HAIR ANALYSIS
**Applications in the Biomedical
and Environmental Sciences**

HAIR ANALYSIS
Applications in the Biomedical and Environmental Sciences

S. A. Katz
A. Chatt

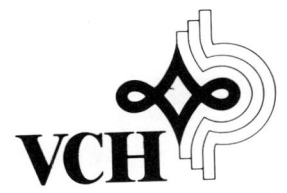

Amares Chatt
Trace Analysis Research Centre
Life Sciences Building
Halifax, Nova Scotia B3H 4J1
CANADA

Sidney A. Katz
Camden College of Arts and Sciences
Rutgers University
Camden, NJ 08102
UNITED STATES

Library of Congress Cataloging-in-Publication Data

Katz, Sidney A., 1935-
   Hair analysis.

   Bibliography: p.
   Includes index.
   1. Hair-Analysis. I. Chatt, A. (Amares) II. Title.
RB47.5.K38   1988   615.9'07   88-33812
ISBN 0-89573-310-2

© 1988 VCH Publishers, Inc.

This work is subject to copyright.

All rights are reserved, whether the whole or part of the material is concerned, specifically those of translation, reprinting, re-use of illustrations, broadcasting, reproduction by photocopying machine or similar means, and storage in data banks.

Registered names, trademarks, etc. used in this book, even when not specifically marked as such, are not to be considered unprotected by law.

Printed in the United States of America.

ISBN 0-89573-310-2 VCH Publishers
ISBN 3-527-26787-5 VCH Verlagsgesellschaft

Distributed in North America by:

VCH Publishers, Inc.
220 East 23rd St., Suite 909
New York, NY 10010

Distributed Worldwide by:

VCH Verlagsgesellschaft
P.O. Box 1260/1280
D-6940 Weinheim
Federal Republic of Germany

In Memoriam

BERNICE JACOBSON CHATT

1947–1987

Preface

During the past three decades, the determination of trace element levels in hair has been a subject of continual interest in the biomedical and environmental sciences. The significance of such measurements as indices for assessing nutritional status, diagnosing diseases, identifying systemic intoxication, and/or monitoring environmental exposures remains, however, the object of much controversy. On the one hand, hair can be considered to be an excretory product, the trace element contents of which reflect mineral metabolism in the body. On the other hand, the origin of the trace elements in hair can be endogenous and/or exogenous, and, therefore, their concentrations bear little relation to the levels in other tissues. While several laboratories have reported firm correlations between the levels of some trace elements in hair and specific environmental or physiological conditions, the lack of standard procedures and the uncertainties about the mechanisms by which the trace elements are incorporated into the hair have precluded generally accepting, in principle, the utility of such analyses. Recently, the Hair Analysis Standards Board of the American Society of Elemental Testing Laboratories and the International Atomic Energy Agency's coordinated research programs on hair analysis have prepared voluntary guidelines in lieu of regulatory standards. These, coupled with the continuing research activities in laboratories throughout the world, can resolve some of these issues and can provide clear guidance on the validity of hair analysis. In this respect, *Hair Analysis: Applications in the Biomedical and Environmental Sciences* has brought together the pros and cons of this technique, and, where applicable, it has made recommendations on its suitability.

Hair Analysis: Applications in the Biomedical and Environmental Sciences includes both the theory and the practice of using hair as a biopsy tissue for trace elements. The various proposals for the biological incorporation of trace elements into the hair are presented, and the external factors possibly affecting the trace element contents of hair are reviewed. Present and past utilizations of hair trace element levels as they relate to nutritional status, disease, heavy metal poisoning, and/or environmental exposure are examined in depth, and methodologies for the collection and preparation of hair samples and for the determination of their trace element contents are given in detail.

In preparing *Hair Analysis: Applications in the Biomedical and Environmental Sciences,* the authors have relied heavily on the open literature, personal communications from colleagues, and their own long-standing interest in the determination of trace elements in hair. Some relevant reports are undoubtedly inadvertently omitted from this work. For this, apologies are offered, and reprints of the omitted material, with appropriate references, are respectfully requested.

Contents

1. The Biological Basis for Trace Elements in Hair   1
   1.1. Historical Introduction   1
   1.2. Hair Morphology, Histologic Structure, and Growth   6
   1.3. Incorporation of Trace Elements into the Hair   10
   1.4. Fundamental Assumptions   14

2. Factors Affecting the Trace Element Contents of Hair   17
   2.1. Length of Hair   17
   2.2. Anatomical Location   19
   2.3. Age, Race, and Gender of Donor   20
   2.4. Hair Color   23
   2.5. Geographical Habitat   24
   2.6. Use of Dietary Supplements and Medicines   25

3. Assessment of Nutritional Status   27
   3.1. Essential Trace Elements   27
   3.2. Manifestations of Mineral Deficiencies   28
   3.3. Applications in Human and Animal Nutrition   31

4. Identification of Systemic Intoxication   37
   4.1. The Toxic Elements   37
   4.2. Clinical Observations   39
   4.3. Relationships between Toxic Elements in Hair and Their Concentrations in Fluids and Other Tissues   41
   4.4. Applications to the Recognition of Acute Chronic Poisoning in Humans   44

5. Diagnosis of Diseases   49
   5.1. Role of Trace Elements in Disease   49
   5.2. Correlations of Disease with Hair Trace Element Levels   51
   5.3. Applications as Diagnostic Aids   60

6. Evaluation of Environmental Exposures   61
   6.1. Occupational Exposures   61
   6.2. Nonoccupational Exposures   65

7. Collection and Preparation of Hair Samples   73
   7.1. Anatomical-Longitudinal Variations of Trace Elements in Hair   73
   7.2. Recommended Sampling Protocols   75
   7.3. Washing Procedures for Removing Exogenous Trace Elements   77
   7.4. Recommended Cleaning Procedures   80
   7.5. Procedures for Dissolving Hair Samples   82

8. Determination of Trace Element Levels in Hair   85
   8.1. Neutron Activation Analysis (NAA)   85
   8.2. Atomic Absorption Spectrometry (AAS)   87
   8.3. Proton-Induced X-Ray Emission (PIXE) Spectrometry   90
   8.4. Other Methods   92
   8.5. Selection of Analytical Techniques   94

9. Quality Assurance of Hair Analysis   95
   9.1. Sampling   96
   9.2. Analysis   96
   9.3. Instrument Calibration   98
   9.4. Quality Control   99
   9.5. Reference Materials   100

10. The Significance of Hair Analysis   105
   10.1. Current Status   105
   10.2. Future Perspectives   112
   10.3. Conclusions   114

References   115

Index   131

1

The Biological Basis for Trace Elements in Hair

Frequent criticisms of some early works on the use of hair as a biopsy tissue for trace elements were based on the lack of information about the mechanisms by which incorporation took place and on the difficulties associated with differentiating between endogenous and exogenous deposition. Subsequent research has addressed these issues, but comprehensive resolutions have not yet been achieved. It is, however, now possible to successfully employ hair analysis if due considerations are directed to the potential problems arising from these unanswered questions.

1.1. Historical Introduction

Many of the early reports credit Flesch (1) with suggesting the use of hair as a biopsy material for trace elements in the body. In 1945, he proposed that hair could function as a minor excretory organ for arsenic and possibly for other toxic elements. That hair might be a metabolic end product, the trace element composition of which reflected the medium from which it was formed, stimulated many of the initial research projects.

Among the more novel applications were the investigations of the arsenic concentrations in Napoleon's hair (2, 3). The results of neutron activation analysis (NAA) on both intact and segmented hair samples indicated repeated exposure to arsenic. This conclusion was reached by assuming an irreversible binding of the arsenic to the hair deep in the follicle, followed by the outward growth of the hair filament at a rate of 0.35 mm/day. The idea of using hair as a recording filament for identifying heavy metal poisoning has subsequently been employed by Giovanoli-Jakubczak and Berg (4). They measured the mercury concentrations in 1-cm segments of bundled hair samples from Iraqi villagers suspected of eating bread made from a grain contaminated with a mercurial fungicide. These measurements were then used to trace the history and extent of the exposure to mercury.

The measurement of arsenic and mercury concentrations in hair has been useful in identifying heavy metal poisoning. Hair, according to Hammer et al. (5), may better reflect the total body pool of some elements than either blood or urine. In this respect, hair could prove to be a practical dosimeter for monitoring elemental environmental pollutants. The International Atomic Energy Agency (IAEA) has coordinated research on the analysis of pollutants in human hair since 1975, and it has stressed the need to establish standard procedures for the collection and preparation of the samples (6). A wide range of environments have been investigated. Lenihan, Smith, and Harvey (7) have used hair analysis to monitor mercury hazards in the occupational environment of the dental profession, and Chattopadhyay, Roberts, and Jervis (8) have used scalp hair as a monitor of community exposure to lead. In the former study, it was proposed that the mercury concentrations of scalp hair were influenced largely by environmental contamination and that the mercury concentrations in pubic hair are determined by mercury ingestion and metabolism. In the latter investigation, a reasonably good blood-lead to hair-lead correlation was obtained for individuals who appeared to be in a steady state with respect to intake and excretion of lead.

Strain et al. (9) extended the use of hair as an indicator of elemental stores in the body to the assessment of zinc nutritional status. They found that the concentration of zinc in the hair of Egyptian dwarfs having zinc deficiency syndrome averaged 54.1 ± 5.5 ppm, while that from normal Egyptians gave a value of 103.3 ± 4.4 ppm. After 2 months of oral zinc sulfate therapy, 30 mg t.i.d., the zinc concentrations in the hair from the dwarfs increased to 121 ± 4.8 ppm. From these studies, they concluded that hair analysis appeared to be a reliable method of assessing body zinc stores.

Klevay (10) studied the zinc concentrations in the hair of Panamanian subjects and concluded that if hair is to be used as a biopsy material for the purpose of comparing zinc nurtiture of individuals or groups, only age-matched individuals or groups may be compared. Deeming and Weber (11) found that hair zinc analysis can be used to aid in the diagnosis of a deficiency or to evaluate dietary intake for the rat, but it cannot be used to assess the state of zinc metabolism. Gershoff et al. (12), on the other hand, concluded from their animal experiments that, except for very special situations, the use of hair trace mineral analyses is of limited or no value in nutritional studies. Chittleborough and Steel (13) have reported no significant increase in hair zinc concentrations after 2 months of oral zinc supplementation, 50 mg q.i.d., to one well-nourished, adult male.

The apparent success of using hair analysis to detect both deficiency and excess of trace elements in the body has been applied to some research on establishing relationships between their concentrations and disease. For example, it is well known that chromium is involved in glucose tolerance (14). Hambidge et al. (15) have shown that the concentration of chromium in the hair of diabetic children is significantly below that of normal children: The respective geometric means were 0.65 and 0.85 ppm. Benjanuvatra and Bennion (16) have reported a similar study on adult victims of this disease. The mean hair chromium concentration of the adult diabetics was 0.094 ppm, whereas that of the control group was 0.241 ppm. While both studies clearly demonstrate depressed chromium concentrations in the hair of the diabetics relative to the respective control groups, there appears to be little agreement on the normal value for chromium in hair. In this respect, the compilation of values for the elemental composition of human tissues by Iyenger, Kollmer, and Bowen (17) lists 0.77, 0.85, 0.55, 0.13, 3.30, 3.25, 3.65, 3.10, and 3.20 ppm under the values for the concentration of chromium in human hair.

It is perhaps the wide divergence of values reported for the normal individual that has hindered the total acceptance of hair analysis as a diagnostic tool. While the concentration of a given trace element in normal blood plasma or in normal blood serum varies within relatively narrow limits, great variations are found in the values reported for the normal hair concentrations. For example, Versieck and Cornelis (18) have reviewed many publications dealing with trace elements in blood and found that most, 31 of 36, reported plasma or serum copper concentrations were in the range of from 0.85 to 1.23 mg/L. A similar review of the literature on the concentrations of trace elements in human hair (19) revealed a range of from 9.1 to 49.8 mg/kg for the average copper contents. When compared to the normal values of trace elements in internal tissues such as blood, the concentrations reported for hair may also be influenced by external contamination. The great variations in the values reported for the normal hair concentrations of trace elements have also been attributed to differences in the experimental procedures used to collect and prepare the samples (20, 21).

Another aspect of hair analysis that has raised questions about its applicability as a diagnostic tool are the reports of increasing concentration gradients for some elements in progressing from the proximal to the distal end of the hair shaft. Hambidge (22) has observed such increases in hair copper concentrations. He interpreted the higher copper concentrations in that part of the hair shaft that has been exposed to the external environment for the longest duration as suggestive of exogenous copper contributing to the total amount determined. Similarly, Kopito and Schwachman (23) have reported that the average lead concentration in the proximal 1.5 cm of the hair shaft was approximately half that of the distal portion (40 ± 43 mg/kg and 76 ± 54 mg/kg, respectively). While recognizing the difficulties in differentiating between endogenous and exogenous lead, they maintain that hair analysis is a reliable means of identifying increased lead burden if sample collection and preparation procedures are standardized, and if carefully matched controls are selected. Valkovic, Rendic, and Phillips (24) have also observed marked increases in the concentrations of lead, as well as those of nickel and arsenic, with increasing distances from the scalp. They attributed these increases to exogenous deposition, and they utilized these measurements for information on exposure to different elemental pollutants.

Despite a quarter century of controversy, the measurement of trace element concentrations in hair remains an area of continuing interest and active research. It has been the subject of at least four books (25, 26, 27, 28), three symposia (29, 30, 31), several reviews, and numerous papers. The apparent conflicts probably result from the failure of some early investigators to develop standard procedures for collecting and preparing the hair samples. In the haste to produce data on the applications of hair analysis, some basic research on the significance of such measurements and on the fundamental principles governing the incorporation of trace elements into the hair may have been neglected. Some corrective steps have been taken (32), and the possible significance of some measurements have been documented. The possible significance of these measurements are summarized in Table 1.1.

Table 1.1 ▪ Possible Significance of Measuring Trace Element Concentrations in Hair

Element	Possible significance of concentration in hair	Reference
Aluminum	May reflect environmental exposure	T-1
Antimony	Elevated levels may reflect occupational exposure and/or systemic intoxication	T-2, T-3
Arsenic	Elevated levels may reflect systemic intoxication	T-4, T-5, T-6, T-7, T-8, T-9
Cadmium	Elevated levels may reflect systemic intoxication	T-10, T-11, T-12
Calcium	Levels may be related to cystic fibrosis, myocardial infarction, and/or nutritional status	T-13, T-14, T-15
Chromium	Levels may be related to diabetes mellitus	T-16, T-17
Cobalt	Unknown	T-18
Copper	Levels may reflect nutritional status	T-19, T-20
Fluorine	Elevated levels may reflect environmental exposure and/or systemic intoxication	T-21
Iodine	Unknown	T-22
Iron	Unknown	T-23
Lead	Elevated levels may reflect systemic intoxication	T-24, T-25, T-26, T-27, T-28, T-29
Lithium	Unknown	T-30
Magnesium	Depressed bound magnesium may be related to cystic fibrosis	T-31
Manganese	Elevated levels may reflect occupational exposure	T-32, T-33
Mercury	Elevated levels may reflect environmental exposures and/or systemic intoxication	T-34, T-35, T-36, T-37, T-38, T-39, T-40, T-41
Molybdenum	Unknown	T-42
Nickel	Elevated levels may reflect environmental exposure	T-43, T-44
Phosphorus	Unknown	T-45
Potassium	Elevated levels may be related to cystic fibrosis or celiac disease	T-46, T-47
Selenium	Elevated levels may reflect occupational or environmental exposures; depressed levels may be related to Keshan disease or multiple sclerosis	T-48, T-49, T-50
Sodium	Elevated levels may be related to cystic fibrosis or celiac disease	T-51, T-52
Zinc	Depressed levels may be related to nutritional deficiency	T-53, T-54, T-55

(*continued*)

Table 1.1 • (Continued)

T-1.	Yokel, R. A., Clin. Chem., 1983, 28, 662–665.
T-2.	Tomza, U., Janicki, T., and Kossman, S., Radiochem. Radioanal. Letters, 1983, 58, 209–220.
T-3.	Lanzel, E., J. Radioanal. Chem., 1980, 58, 347–357.
T-4.	Olguin, A., Jauge, P., Cebrian, M., and Albores, A., Proc. West. Pharmacol. Soc., 1983, 26, 175–177.
T-5.	Leslie, A. C. D., and Smith, H., Arch. Toxicol., 1978, 41, 163–167.
T-6.	Valentine, J. L., Kang, H. K., and Spivey, G., Environ. Res., 1979, 20, 24–32.
T-7.	Obrusnik, I., and Bencko, V., Radiochem. Radioanal. Letters, 1979, 38, 189–196.
T-8.	Baker, E. L., Hayes, C. G., Landrigan, P. J., Handke, J. L., Leger, R. T., Housworth, W. J., and Harrington, J. M., Amer. J. Epidem., 1977, 106, 261–273.
T-9.	See T-3.
T-10.	Milosevic, M., Petrovic, L., Petrovic, D., and Pejuskovic, B., Arch. Hig. Rada Toksikol., 1980, 31, 209–217.
T-11.	Kollmer, W., Sci. Total Environ., 1982, 25, 41–51.
T-12.	Menzel, N., and Wittmaack, K., in *Trace Element Analytical Chemistry in Medicine and Biology, Vol. 2*, P. Bratter and P. Schramel, eds., Walter de Gruyter and Co., Berlin, 1983, pp. 1002–1008.
T-13.	Kopito, L., Elian, E., and Shwachman, H., Pediatrics, 1972, 49, 620–624.
T-14.	Bacsò, J., Kovàcs, P., and Horvàth, S., Radiochem. Radioanal. Letters, 1978, 33, 273–280.
T-15.	Perkons, A., Velandia, J., and Dienes, M., J. Forens. Sci., 1977, 22, 95–105.
T-16.	Hambidge, K. M., Diabetes, 1968, 17, 517–519.
T-17.	Hunt, A. E., Ph.D. Thesis, Colorado State University, Ft. Collins, 1983.
T-18.	Coleman, R., Harrington, J., and Seales, J., Brit. Med. J., 1973, 1, 527–529.
T-19.	Krishnamachari, K., Amer. J. Clin. Nutr., 1974, 27, 108–111.
T-20.	Gregor, J., Amer. J. Clin. Nutr., 1978, 31, 269–275.
T-21.	Weisener, W., Goerner, W., and Niese, S., in *Nuclear Activation Techniques in the Life Sciences, 1978*, International Atomic Energy Agency, Vienna, 1979, pp. 307–320.
T-22.	Ganor, S., Gedalia, I., and Brand, N., J. Invest. Dermatol., 1964, 43, 5–6.
T-23.	Izumi, K., Tokyo Ika Daizaku Zasshi, 1983, 41, 43–49.
T-24.	Marzulli, F. N., Watlington, P. M., and Maibach, H. I., Curr. Prob. Dermatol., 1978, 7, 196–204.
T-25.	Clayton, E., and Wooller, K. K., IEEE Trans. Nuc. Sci., 1983, NS-30, 1326–1328.
T-26.	Niculescu, T., Dumitru, R., Botha, V., Alexandrescu, R., and Manolescu, N., Brit. J. Indust. Med., 1983, 40, 67–70.
T-27.	Jervis, R. E., Tiefenbach, B., and Chattopadhyay, A., J. Radioanal. Chem., 1977, 37, 751–760.
T-28.	See T-10.
T-29.	Kopito, L., Byers, R. K., and Shwachman, H., New England J. Med., 1967, 276, 949–953.
T-30.	Rimland, B., and Larson, G. E., J. Learning Disabilities, 1983, 16, 1–8.
T-31.	See T-13.
T-32.	Sakurai, S., J. Iwate Med. Assoc., 1980, 32, 869–884.
T-33.	Akashi, J., Fukushima, I., Imahori, A., Shiobara, S., Takahashi, Y., and Tomura, K., J. Radioanal. Chem., 1982, 68, 59–65.
T-34.	Lin, S. M., Chiang, C. H., Tseng, C. L., and Yang, M. H., Radiochem. Radioanal. Letters, 1982, 56, 261–272.
T-35.	Lodenius, M., and Seppänen, H., Chemosphere, 1982, 11, 755–759.
T-36.	Hansen, J. C., Wulf, H. C., Kromann, N., and Alboge, K., Sci. Total Environ., 1983, 26, 233–243.

(continued)

Table 1.1 ▪ (*Continued*)

T-37.	Kyle, J. H., and Ghani, N., Sci. Total Environ., 1983, 26, 157–162.
T-38.	Cigna, L., Clemente, G. F., and Santaroni, G., Arch. Environ. Health, 1976, 31, 160–165.
T-39.	Biso, J. M., Cohen, I. M., and Resnizky, S. M., Radiochem. Radioanal. Letters, 1983, 58, 175–180.
T-40.	Sherlock, J. C., Lindsay, D. G., Hislop, J. E., Evans, W. H., and Collier, T. R., Arch. Environ. Health, 1982, 37, 271–278.
T-41.	Pritchard, J. G., McMullin, J. F., and Sikondari, A. H., Brit. Dent. J., 1982, November 2, 333–336.
T-42.	See T-30.
T-43.	Spruit, D., and Bongaarte, P. J. M., in *Clinical Chemistry and Clinical Toxicology of Metals*, S. S. Brown, ed., Elsevier/North Holland Biomedical Press, Amsterdam, 1977, pp. 261–264.
T-44.	Hagedorn-Götz, H., Kuppers, G., and Stoeppler, M., Arch. Toxicol., 1977, 38, 275–285.
T-45.	Bland, J., John J. Bastyr College of Naturopathic Med., 1979, 1, 3–6.
T-46.	See T-13.
T-47.	Kopito, L., and Shwachman, H., in *First Human Hair Symposium*, A. C. Brown, ed., Medcom Press, New York, 1974, pp. 83–90.
T-48.	Yang, G., Wang, S., Zhou, R., and Sun, S., Amer. J. Clin. Nutr., 1983, 37, 872–881.
T-49.	Yang, G., Wang, G., Yin, T., Sun, S., Zhou, R., Man, R., Zhai, F., Guo, S., Wang, H-Z., and You, D., Acta Nutrimenta Sinica, 1982, 4, 191–200.
T-50.	Wang, M-Y., Acta Nutrimenta Sinica, 1982, 4, 201–207.
T-51.	See T-13.
T-52.	See T-47.
T-53.	Rielly, C., Proc. Nutr. Soc. Australia, 1981, 6, 141–143.
T-54.	Reinhold, J., Amer. J. Clin. Nutr., 1966, 16, 294–300.
T-55.	Hambidge, K. M., and Silverman, A., Arch. Dis. Child., 1973, 48, 567.

1.2. Hair Morphology, Histologic Structure, and Growth

The hair shaft is a keratinized filament that is formed from the matrix cells at the bottom of the hair follicle deep in the epidermal epithelium. Each follicle is a miniature organ that contains both muscular and glandular components. A diagram of an active human hair follicle is presented in Figure 1.1. The hair filament in the diagram has been divided into three zones along its axis. The innermost zone at and around the bulb of the hair is the site of biological synthesis and organization. The next zone in the outward direction along the hair shaft is the zone of keratinization (keratogenous zone), where the hair fiber undergoes hardening or solidification through cystine cross-linking. The final zone is the region of permanent hair. It consists of dehydrated and cornified cells and the intercellular binding material.

Cross sections of the human hair shaft usually show three types of cells. These are apparent in Figure 1.2. The outermost region of cells, those of the cuticle, form the outer protective layer around the hair fiber. The cuticle surrounds the cells of the cortex, which makes up the major part of the hair shaft. The most central region of the hair shaft contains the cells of the medulla.

The cuticle consists of flat, overlapping cells. Each cell is from 0.5×10^{-4} to 1.0×10^{-4} cm thick and approximately 45×10^{-4} cm long. In human hair, the

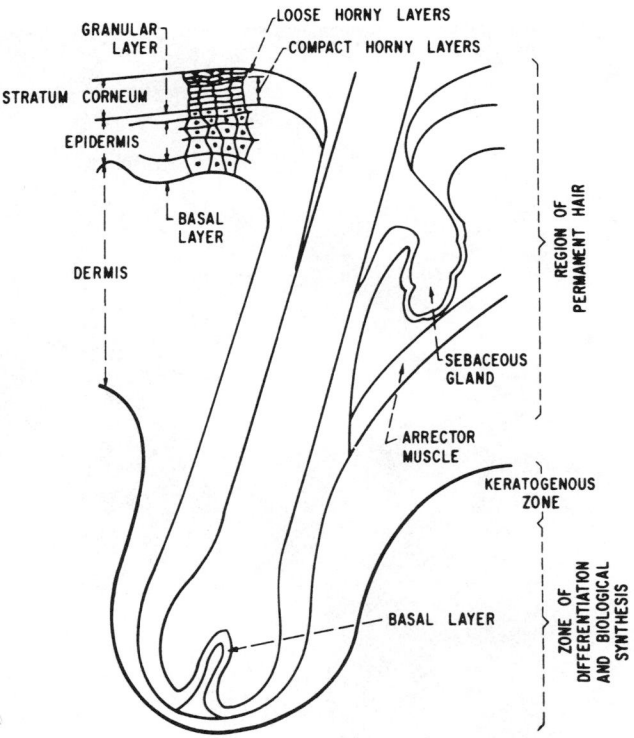

Figure 1.1 ■ A hair follicle with its fiber, as the fiber emerges from the scalp. [From C. R. Robbins, *Chemical and Physical Behavior of Human Hair*. New York: Van Nostrand. Reprinted by permission.]

cuticle is from 5 to 10 cell layers thick. The cells of the cortex are from 1.0×10^{-4} to 6.0×10^{-4} cm in thickness and approximately 100×10^{-4} cm in length. Spindle-shaped, fibrous microfilaments (0.1×10^{-4} to 0.4×10^{-4} cm in diameter) are dispersed throughout the cells of the cortex. The cells of the medulla are unorganized and loosely packed. During dehydration, they shrivel up and leave a series of vacuoles along the central axis of the hair shaft.

Human hair consists of approximately 80% protein and 15% water, with smaller amounts of lipid and inorganic materials. The amino acid composition of the hair protein, although subject to variations due to factors such as genetics, diet, illness or wellness, weathering, cosmetic treatment, environment, and so on, has been extensively studied. Typical values, as reported by Robbins (33), are listed in Table 1.2. The water content of hair varies directly with the ambient relative humidity. Some values are presented in Table 1.3. The lipid material in the hair ranges from 1% to 9%. This material is derived from sebum and consists of free fatty acids; mono-, di-, and triglycerides; wax esters; hydrocarbons; and alcohols. The mineral content of hair is from 0.25% to 0.95%, on a dry ash basis.

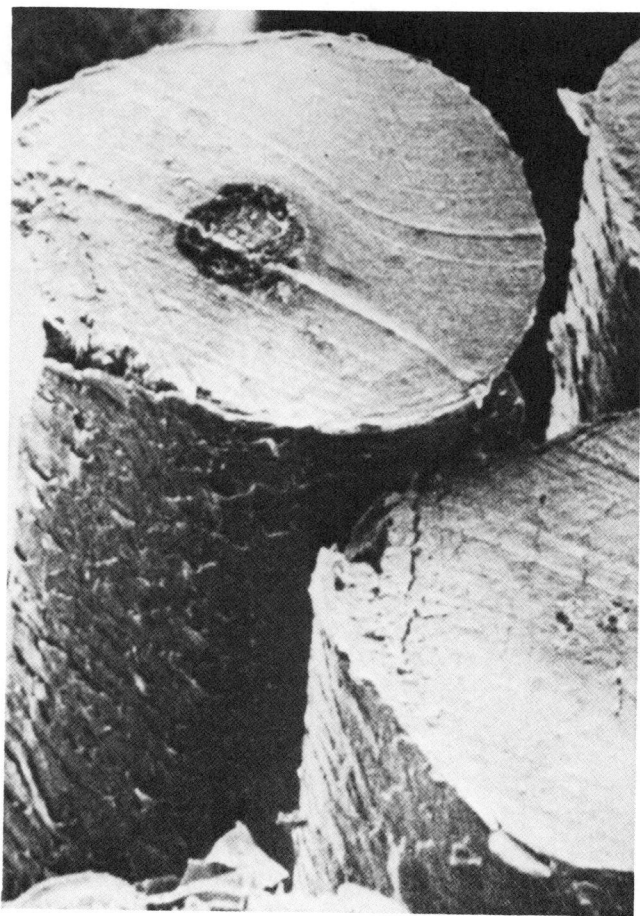

Figure 1.2 ▪ Cross-section of human hair showing cuticle, cortex, and medulla.

The sebaceous gland develops from the follicular epithelium. The secretion of this gland, sebum, diffuses into the canal of the follicle and flows out to impregnate the hair shaft. The apocrine sweat gland also develops from the epithelium of the hair follicle, and its duct opens into the canal just above the connection with the sebaceous gland. The eccrine sweat glands are distributed over the entire skin surface. They are derived from the surface epithelium. Hopps (34) has identified sebum and sweat as possible sources of the trace elements found in the permanent hair.

The hair follicle does not produce hair continuously. Periods of activity alternate with periods of rest. Characteristic changes in the hair follicle and hair shaft accompany the cycle. This hair cycle is divided into three stages:

Table 1.2 ▪ Amino Acid Composition of Human Hair[a]

Amino acid	Micromoles per gram of dry hair
Alanine	362–384
Arginine	499–550
Aspartic acid	444–453
Cysteic acid	22–40
Glutamic acid	995–1036
Glycine	463–513
Half cystine	1407–1512
Histidine	64–86
Isoleucine	244–255
Lecuine	502–529
Lysine	206–222
Methionine	50–56
Phenylalanine	132–149
Proline	646–708
Serine	1013–1091
Threonine	648–673
Tyrosine	177–195
Valine	477–513

[a]According to Robbins (33).

1. The *anagen stage*, during which active growth takes place
2. The *catagen stage*, which is a transitional phase characterized by cessation of active proliferation and the formation of "club hairs"
3. The *telogen* or resting *stage*.

The onset of anagen is accompanied by increased metabolic activity of the matrix cells just above the papilla at the bottom of the follicle. A fine strand extends downward and envelops the papilla, and the bottom of the follicle is pushed more deeply into the dermis by continual cell division. The new hair begins as a thin filament pushing its way upward into the follicular canal. The cells of the developing hair undergo differentiation to cuticle, cortex, and medulla, and the keratiniza-

Table 1.3 ▪ Water Content of Human Hair

Relative humidity at 20°C (%)	Water content (%)
29.2	6.0
40.3	7.6
50.0	9.8
65.0	12.8
70.3	13.6

tion process is initiated. While this complex series of events is not fully defined, it is possible that at this point, the endogenous trace elements, some of which may be complexed with protein, are incorporated into the hair from the metabolic milieu of the matrix cells, together with the contributions from connective tissue of the papilla, circulating blood and lymph, and other intra- and extracellular fluids (35). The developing hair becomes fully keratinized, and it is ultimately extruded through the skin as a permanent hair.

During the growth phase, the follicles of the scalp produce hair at a rate of from 0.2 to 0.5 mm/day. Some of the growth rates quoted for scalp hair as well as for other anatomical sites are summarized in Table 1.4. These growth rates and the duration of follicular activity appear to be highly variable and dependent upon such factors as age, race, gender, anatomical location, season, and so on. The length of the hair cycle and its component stages have been studied by Saitoh, Uzuka, and Sakamoto (36). Their results and the results of others are presented in Table 1.5.

In the catagen stage, the actively growing hair undergoes transformation into a dead club hair. The matrix cells differentiate into those of the internal root sheath and those of the hair shaft. The bottommost matrix cells degenerate, and the production of new cells for the internal root sheath ceases. Simultaneously, the matrix cells become separated from the connective tissue of the papilla, and they form a short column of epithelial cells. The lowermost end of the disconnected hair shaft becomes fully keratinized and forms the dry, white node characteristic of a club hair.

The formation of club hairs reflects the telogen stage. Club hairs are often retained in the upper portion of the follicular canal at the level of the arrector pili attachment. While the metabolic activity of the follicle ceases during telogen, the trace element contents of the club hair may reflect the metabolic milieu of the preceding anagen.

1.3. Incorporation of Trace Elements into the Hair

Thirty years ago, Flesch (1) identified the permanent hair as a unique medium for studying the excretion of heavy metals from the body, on the basis of permanent hair's long life span, keratinous structure, and metabolic inertness. He recognized the difficulty in establishing whether or not poisoning had taken place, based on the ability of keratin to combine with heavy metals from internal as well as from external sources. In this respect, Hopps (34) has proposed six possible sources of trace elements:

1. Those taken up by the matrix during histogenesis
2. Those deposited from sebum
3. Those sorbed or otherwise transferred to the hair from eccrine sweat
4. Those simultaneously incorporated into the permanent hair from apocrine sweat
5. Those deposited from the external environment after the hair has been extruded through the skin

Table 1.4 ■ Hair Growth Rates

Anatomical site	Rate	Reference
Pubis	0.2 mm/day	T-56
Unspecified	1 cm/month	T-57
Scalp	0.4 mm/day	T-58
Scalp	10 mm/month	T-59
Scalp	1 cm/month	T-60
Scalp	0.2–0.5 mm/day	T-61
Axilla	0.3–0.4 mm/day	T-61
Beard	0.2 mm/day	T-61
Scalp	0.75–1.12 mm/day	T-62
Scalp	1.1 ± 0.2 mm/day	T-63
Scalp	0.7–1.1 cm/month	T-64
Scalp (children)	10.0–13.5 mm/month	T-65
Scalp (adults)	7.1–12.0 mm/month	T-65
Scalp	0.35 mm/day	T-66
Scalp	1.0–1.5 cm/month	T-67

T-56. Dang, H. S., Jaiswal, D. D., Mehta, U., and Deshpande, A., Sci. Total Environ., 1983, 31, 187–192.

T-57. Grodzins, A., Trans. New York Acad. Sci., 1980, 40, 93–98.

T-58. Katz, S. A., and Wood, J. D., Chem. Internat., 1980, 6, 12–15.

T-59. Toribara, T. Y., and Jackson, D. A., Clin. Chem., 1982, 28, 650–654.

T-60. Hambidge, K. M., Franklin, M. L., and Jacobs, M. A., Amer. J. Clin. Nutr., 1972, 25, 380–383.

T-61. Hopps, H. C., Sci. Total Environ., 1977, 7, 71–89.

T-62. Giovanoli-Jakubczak, T., and Berg, G. C., Arch. Environ. Health, 1974, 28, 139–144.

T-63. Chattopadhyay, A., Roberts, T. M., and Jervis, R. E., Arch. Environ. Health, 1977, Sept./Oct., 226–236.

T-64. Leslie, A. C. D., and Smith, H., Arch. Toxicol., 1978, 41, 163–167.

T-65. Kopito, L., Byers, R. K., and Shwachman, H., New England J. Med., 1967, 276, 949–953.

T-66. Smith, H., Forshufvud, S., and Wassen, A., Nature, 1962, 194, 725–726.

T-67. Airey, D., Environ. Health Prospec., 1983, 52, 303–316.

6. Those from cosmetic and/or pharmaceutical preparations applied to the scalp or other body surfaces.

Chittleborough (35) and Rivlin (37) have also suggested sweat, environmental contamination, and previous beauty treatments as potential exogenous sources of trace elements in the hair.

Table 1.5 ▪ Duration of Stages in the Human Hair Cycle

Anatomical site	Anagen	Catagen	Telogen	Total	Reference
Scalp	900 days	Several days	100 days	1000 days	T-68
Scalp	—	—	—	16–20 months	T-69
Beard	4–11 months	—	10–75 days	7–11 months	T-69
Pubes	11–18 months	—	12–17 months	—	T-69
Scalp	3–6 months	—	2 months	5–8 months	T-70

T-68. Hopps, H. C., Sci. Total Environ., 1977, 7, 71–89.
T-69. Flesch, P., in *Physiology and Biochemistry of the Skin*, S. Rothman, ed., University of Chicago Press, Chicago, 1954, pp. 601–661.
T-70. Saitoh, M., Uzuka, M., and Sakamoto, M., J. Invest. Dermatol., 1970, 54, 65–81.

To differentiate between endogenous and exogenous trace elements, most laboratories include some kind of cleaning procedure in the analytical scheme to remove surface contamination. Such differentiation is necessary when the results of the analysis are used to assess nutritional status, diagnose diseases, and/or identify heavy-metal poisoning.

1.3.1. Endogenous Trace Elements

The endogenous trace elements are those incorporated into the hair at the root during anagen. It has not been demonstrated that such incorporations reflect random uptake from either the metabolic milieu or a biologically regulated synthetic process, or both.

As evidence of endogenous deposition, Ryabukhin (14) cites high levels of mercury in the hair of Iraqi peasants who had ingested grain treated with a mercurial fungicide and the above-normal hair mercury levels of some residents of the Netherlands who had consumed mercury-contaminated fish. Airey (38) has also observed a positive correlation between hair mercury levels and the consumption of mercury-contaminated fish. In her excellent review on the subject (39), she presents convincing evidence to support a direct relationship between mercury ingestion and mercury levels in the hair. In a well-controlled animal experiment, Berg and Kollmer (40) have clearly demonstrated that radiotracer mercury administered either by intravenous injection or by gastric intubation was partially excreted in the hair. Hansen *et al.* (41) have, in addition, reported a firm correlation ($r = .9222$) between the concentrations of mercury in hair and blood from Greenlanders who consume large amounts of seal.

Further evidence for endogenous deposition of trace elements in the hair is found in the classic works of Kopito *et al.* (42, 43). They reported elevated lead levels in the hair, blood, and urine of children with clinically confirmed chronic lead poisoning. Similarly, Valentine *et al.* (44) have reported elevated arsenic levels in the hair, blood, and urine of California residents whose drinking water contained 0.4 ppm of arsenic. While it could be argued that the elevated levels of arsenic in the hair reflected the deposition of exogenous arsenic from bathing in the arsenic-contaminated water, the elevated blood and urine levels support, at least partially, endogenous deposition. Reports on selenium intoxication in China (45) also show elevated selenium levels in the hair, blood, and urine. The source of selenium in this case was the food crops from soils rich in this element.

While it appears that ingested toxic elements are endogenously incorporated into the hair, similar evidence for the micronutrients is less convincing. Klevay (10) reported "no correlations were demonstrable between the zinc content of hair and plasma, hair and red blood cells" (p. 287), in a nutritional survey of some 200 Panamanian subjects. He did, however, report a correlation for hair copper and plasma copper (46). Chittleborough and Steel (13) failed to observe an increase in the zinc concentration of facial hair in response to zinc ingestion, and Deeming and Weber (11) found that plasma zinc correlated very poorly with hair zinc in a controlled dietary experiment with 100 rats. In a study involving the administration of both zinc and copper to 200 rats in drinking water, Jacob, Klevay, and Logan (47) found a correlation between the copper levels of hair and liver. but they found no correlations for the corresponding zinc levels. McKenzie (48) measured the zinc levels in hair, blood (serum), and urine of 110 New Zealand adults. She reported "marginally negative correlations" ($p < .05$) between the levels in hair and blood and in hair and urine. Among her subjects were three galvanizers whose hair zinc concentrations were 1160, 2240, and 10,320 ppm, respectively.

1.3.2. Exogenous Trace Elements

The incorporation into the hair of exogenous trace elements can take place under a wide variety of conditions in the occupational, domestic, and recreational environments. While their presence certainly reflects environmental exposure, it also leads to confusion in the interpretation of the analytical results for the (1) identification of systemic intoxication, (2) assessment of nutritional status, and/or (3) diagnosis of disease. Exogenous toxic elements could lead to faulty conclusions regarding heavy-metal poisoning, and the exogenous deposition of those elements recognized as micronutrients could mask their depressed endogenous levels if dietary deficiencies are reflected as such. Depending on the disease–trace-element relationships, providing that they can be determined from hair analysis, exogenous deposition could give a false positive elevation or could mask a depression.

As early as 1965, Bate and Dyer (49) found that less than 50% of the amounts of trace elements exogenously deposited in or on permanent hair was removed by their cleaning procedure, washing with an aqueous solution of a nonionic detergent followed by rinsing with water. Subsequently, Bate (50) reported that exogenously deposited antimony, gold, mercury, and silver were only partially removed from human hair by washing with agents such as $0.1\,N$ nitric acid, $0.1\,N$ ammonia, or $0.1\,M$ EDTA. Gordus (51) has found "that the use of certain prescription scalp medications result in selenium hair levels that are 20 to 40 times higher than normal" (p.

235). Toribara and Jackson (52) observed an increase from 143 to 1970 ppm zinc after human hair was soaked in a solution containing 500 ppm zinc at physiological pH, and Clanet *et al.* (53) reported that simulated toilet and cosmetic treatments increased the copper and zinc contents of human hair tenfold and threefold, respectively, after a so-called "standard" washing procedure. While the use of cosmetic preparations containing toxic elements leads to exogenous deposition, it can also lead to endogenous incorporation. Marzulli and Brown (54) attributed to percutaneous adsorption the elevated mercury levels in the hair, blood, and urine of a female victim of mercury poisoning who had applied an ammoniated mercury skin bleach to her hands and arms for several years. Similarly, the increase in lead concentrations of pubic and axillary hair was attributed to the percutaneous adsorption of lead from a hair dye containing 2% lead acetate (55). After 3 months of daily use, the lead concentrations in hair from the scalp, axilla, and pubes reached levels in excess of 7000, 300, and 400 ppm, respectively.

1.4. Fundamental Assumptions

The literature contains a wide divergence of opinions on the significance of trace element concentrations in hair. Some reports ignore the issue completely and present tabulations of results from various populations (56–59). Others quote earlier works that quoted even earlier works identifying hair as a minor excretory organ, metabolic endproduct, or accumulator tissue (60–63). Some take a stronger position and maintain that the trace element levels of hair reflect a permanent record of the trace element content of the body during the growth phase of the hair (64–68). There are also those that reject the significance of hair analysis for reasons of wide normal ranges and/or exogenous contamination (69, 70). Most recent reports, however, recognize the current uncertainties and difficulties regarding the interpretation of trace element levels in hair and either optimistically look forward to future developments for clarification (71, 72) or urge caution in drawing conclusions from the present data (14, 73).

The simplest model for the incorporation of endogenous trace elements into the hair assumes their passive transfer from the metabolic milieu, under the influence of concentration gradients. The excesses of toxic elements accompanying heavy metal poisoning or the deficiencies of micronutrients associated with dietary insufficiencies are then reflected as deviations from the normal values. Similarly, excesses or deficiencies of trace elements in the metabolic milieu resulting from physiological distress are also reflected as deviations from the normal values.

The sulfhydryls, or (more likely) the disulfides, of the hair protein have been proposed as the binding sites for heavy metals (74–76). The amino groups may also be involved (75). The binding of endogenous trace elements in the fully keratinized hair is assumed to be irreversible, or, at least, quite firm.

While these assumptions are frequently employed to support the significance of hair mineral analysis, they fall short of explaining several observations. For example, Flynn et al. (77) have reported the appearance of ^{65}Zn in the hair within a time as short as 2 hours after administration, but Rabinowitz, Wetherill, and Kopple (78) found a delay of approximately 35 days for the appearance of ^{204}Pb in facial hair. Two hours is far too short a time to be consistent with the assumptions of the simple passive transfer model. Possibly, the ^{65}Zn was partially excreted in the sweat and subsequently deposited in or on the hair as exogenous material within this time. To explain the 35-day delay in the appearance of the ^{204}Pb, multiple exchanges between several pools in the body were assumed rather than simple transfer from blood to hair.

Chittleborough and Steel (13) have expanded upon this pool model by assuming the active transfer of micronutrients—zinc in particular—from pool to pool via multiple equilibria and steady states. A general schematic for their pool model is presented in Figure 1.3. The pool model, the exact form of which varies with the element under consideration, assumes filled pools for essential trace elements under normal conditions. Stresses on the system caused by or resulting in excesses or deficiencies of trace elements are ultimately reflected in their endogenous hair concentrations.

While the pool model shows promise of becoming a viable explanation for the incorporation of trace elements into the hair, it has yet to be experimentally confirmed. For this reason, the Hair Analysis Board (32) has made more conservative assumptions in establishing the clinical utility of trace element concentrations in hair, specifically the following:

1. Tightly bound elements in hair, those not extractable by aqueous solutions,

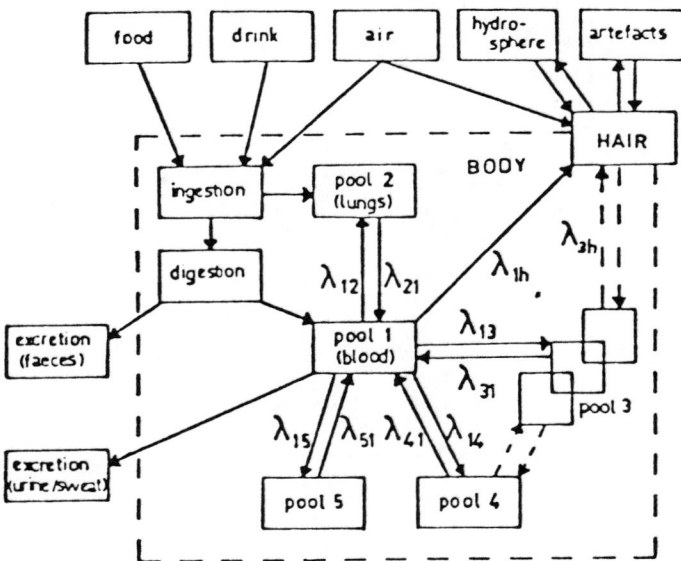

Figure 1.3 ▪ Some pathways for trace elements in the environment via pools in the body.

may be related to their respective metabolic regulations in the biologically active hair tissue
2. Bound elements are considered to be endogenous (i.e., deposited during protein synthesis)
3. Water-soluble elements are considered to be exogenous (i.e., the result of environmental contamination)
4. The hair concentrations of the bound elements may be influenced by factors such as dietary intake, overall nutritional status, endocrine and metabolic functions, age, gender, general health status, and sociological factors
5. Reduced or elevated hair concentrations of an element should not be interpreted as an indicator of nutritional deficiency or toxic excess
6. A clinician must develop expertise and interpretive skills in the application of trace element profiles in hair before using them in patient management
7. Hair analysis is a screening rather than a diagnostic tool; other biomedical parameters and clinical tests must be considered in establishing a diagnosis.

It is in this frame of reference that hair analysis may be applied to biomedical and environmental science. Leyton (78a) has put the use of hair analysis into a proper perspective: He said, "It is essential that hair analysis be regarded as neither a routine procedure nor a diagnostic tool; rather, when undertaken with care it is a useful procedure under certain conditions to confirm or refute clinical indications of toxic metal overburden or nutritional deficiency" (p. 1109).

2

Factors Affecting the Trace Element Contents of Hair

In addition to the lack of a firm theoretical foundation, the significance of trace element concentrations in hair is questioned on the basis of the difficulties associated (1) with differentiating between those of endogenous origin and those deposited exogenously and (2) with rationalizing the wide range of normal values reported in the literature. With respect to the latter, some of the inconsistency can be attributed to differences in sample collection and preparation procedures from laboratory to laboratory. Recent movements to standardize these procedures may lead to better interlaboratory agreement, but factors such as (1) the distance of the sample from the scalp and the anatomical location of the hair sample; (2) the age, race, and gender of the donor; (3) the geographical habitat of the donor; and (4) his or her dietary supplements and medications have also been reported as affecting the trace element contents of hair. The use of age-matched, gender-matched cohorts may produce normal values for specific subgroups of the general population.

2.1. Length of Hair

Exogenous deposition is clearly a major factor for the increasing concentration gradients Hambidge (22) observed for copper in progressing from the proximal to the distal end of the hair. Some of his data are presented graphically in Figure 2.1. None of the subjects used hair dyes or bleaches, and each sample was individually washed in hexane, ethanol, and deionized water, sequentially. From his observations, he concluded (1) that copper from the external environment contributes to the total copper content of the hair and (2) that the most distal part of the hair shaft shows the highest copper concentration because it has been exposed to the external environment for the longest duration. He urges caution in the interpretation of analytical data on hair copper levels, and he recommends that samples should be taken from the recently grown hair within 1–2 cm from the scalp.

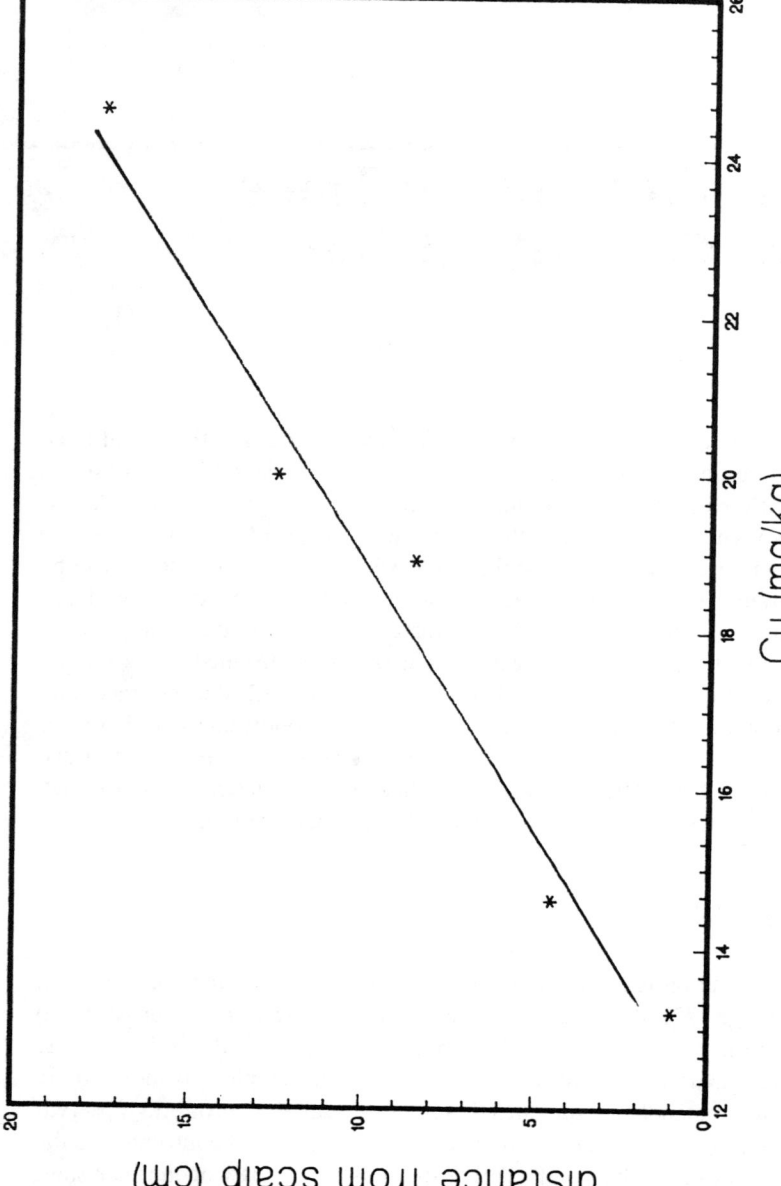

Figure 2.1 ▪ Increasing copper concentrations at increasing distances from the scalp. [After Hambidge (22).]

Kopito and Shwachman (23) reported a significant difference ($p < .001$) between the mean lead values for the proximal 1.5 cm of hair (40 ± 43 mg/kg) and the most distal 1.5 cm of hair (76 ± 54 mg/kg). Of the 22 subjects whose hair was evaluated, only one showed more lead in the proximal end (49 mg/kg) than in the distal end (22 mg/kg). In five subjects, the lead contents of the distal ends were 20 to 50 times greater than in the proximal ends. This differential was attributed to long exposures to environmental factors, such as dust, dirt, sweat, sebum, and environmental sources.

Valkovic et al. (24) have also observed that the concentration of some trace elements in hair increase with increasing distances from the scalp. Their report lacks specifics on the collection and preparation of the samples, and their results are presented relative to zinc. Nonetheless, the ratios of arsenic to zinc and of lead to zinc show a 10-fold increase in progressing from the proximal to the distal end, and the ratio of nickel to zinc similarly shows a 20-fold increase. These increases are attributed to entrance into the hair by deposition onto its surface and by later diffusion into the hair structure. Interestingly, the ratios for iron to zinc and copper to zinc do not show marked increases along the hair. It is quite possible that the arsenic, lead, and nickel reflect a time-dependent exogenous deposition, and that the iron and copper reflect steady-state endogenous deposition.

Arunachalam et al. (79) have also reported data on the concentrations of trace elements in the distal and proximal ends of the hair. The mean values for 35 females show little change for iron and zinc. The concentration of labile elements such as chlorine and potassium, however, are more than 50% less at the distal ends than they are at the proximal ends; that is, chlorine decreased from 2650 to 980 mg/kg, and potassium decreased from 30 to 12 mg/kg. It is possible that repeated washings continually remove the labile elements from the hair.

To compensate for the variations of trace element concentrations along the length of the hair, most laboratories have identified the proximal inch of hair as the best sample for the determination of recently deposited, endogenous trace elements.

2.2. Anatomical Location

Assuming that the processes involved with the endogenous incorporation of trace elements into the hair are uniform over the entire body, samples collected from covered anatomical sites, such as the pubes, should be less vulnerable to exogenous contamination than samples collected from the scalp. Several investigations have attempted to take advantage of this possibility, but results, in some cases, are contradictory.

Chittleborough and Steel (80) have measured zinc, cadmium, lead, and copper concentration in samples of facial and scalp hair collected from the same individual. Their results for six replicate determinations on uniform samples from each anatomical site are summarized in Table 2.1. The concentrations in scalp hair were from 2 to 20 times higher than in facial hair. Although details on the sample collection are not fully described, it is possible that the beard samples were collected daily with an

Table 2.1 ■ Zinc, Cadmium, Lead, and Copper Concentrations in Scalp and Facial Hair of the Same Individual[a]

Anatomical site	Element, mg/kg ± SD			
	Zinc	Cadmium	Lead	Copper
Scalp	521 ± 31	4.9 ± 0.6	8.1 ± 0.4	192 ± 6
Face	172 ± 11	1.9 ± 0.3	4.6 ± 0.1	12 ± 1

[a] After Chittleborough and Steel (80).

electric shaver and pooled, whereas the scalp hair was collected as a single cutting. The latter would then be subject to greater external contamination.

Orlando et al. (81) have reported significant differences ($p < .01$) between the scalp and pubic hair concentrations of lead, iron, copper, and zinc in 39 female subjects. The mean values for these elements were higher in scalp hair. On the other hand, DeAntonio et al. (73), whose work has been criticized for lack of statistical rigor (82), have reported no significant differences between scalp and pubic hair concentrations of calcium, magnesium, copper, iron, and zinc for a population of 20 females and 40 males. More recently, Dang et al. (83) found no significant differences in the concentrations of copper, zinc, and manganese in scalp and pubic hair from 15 normal, nonpregnant subjects.

Rees and Campbell (84) recommend that pubic, axillary, or pectoral hair be sampled to ensure that the results of hair analysis "reflect the conditions of body tissues and not the hair dye or other surface contaminants" (p. 2). Hopps (34), however, has proposed that pubic hair is less suitable than scalp hair because the former grows more slowly and is more vulnerable to contamination by sweat and sebum. While there was no experimental evidence to support this proposal, hair from different parts of the body is certainly exposed to different external conditions with respect to toilet, cosmetics, topical medications, and so on. The potential for differences in exogenous trace elements exists. It would seem, therefore, that until such time as exogenous trace elements can be differentiated from endogenous trace elements, caution should be exercised in pooling data on trace element levels in hair from different anatomical locations.

The advantage of using pubic hair is as a check against misinterpretation of elevated levels in scalp hair as an indication of systemic intoxication. Both Sumie et al. (85) and Lenihan et al. (86) have used this approach to evaluate mercury exposure and intoxication in the dental profession. Scalp hair contained more mercury than did the pubic hair of the subjects in these studies, indicating a significant exogenous contribution to the samples from the former anatomical site.

2.3. Age, Race, and Gender of Donor

The literature contains frequent references to differences in the trace element concentrations of hair from various subgroups of the general population. These differences have been observed between subgroups formed on the basis of age, race, and gender. The changing nutritional requirements and metabolic processes associated with aging may be responsible for differences among age subgroups. The different dietary habits of various cultural groups may be responsible for the differences in hair trace element levels reported for specific racial and ethnic groups, and the differences reported on the basis of gender may be due to the differences in hormonal activity.

The scalp hair concentrations of copper, lead, and cadmium for those under 30 years of age are significantly different from those for the over-40 population (62). The younger group showed higher levels of these elements. Petering et al. (87) found that "zinc in the hair of males increased from 105 ppm at age 2 to 180 ppm at age 12 and thereafter declined slowly to 125 ppm at age 80" (p. 204). Similarly, they found that hair copper levels increased from 13 to 60 ppm and then declined to 10 ppm. Takeuchi et al. (88) have reported that the hair concentrations of chlorine, iodine, aluminum, potassium, vanadium, and manganese decreased with advanced age, while those of magnesium, calcium, copper, and zinc increased with increasing age. The hair mercury concentration was found to show an increasing trend with age by Imahori et al. (89). Mean hair lead concentrations, on the other hand, did not show significant differences for the age groupings of 1–21, 22–42, 43–87 years (90). Creason et al. (91) have, however, found that the scalp-hair lead concentrations decreased rapidly with age for 1- to 15-year-old female children. Eads and Lambdin (61), however, observed "a trend of increasing lead content with age" (p. 249) for males. The reverse trend, a decline from 25 mg lead per kg of hair at age 2 years to 10 mg lead per kg of hair at age 85, was reported by Petering et al. (92).

Clearly, the literature is contradictory on the effect of age of the donor and the lead content of hair. There is, however, an abundance of evidence to support the variation in hair trace element contents with age. In this respect, Klevay's (10) conclusion—"if hair is to be used as a biopsy material . . . only age matched individuals or groups may be compared" (p. 288)—is indeed valid.

Differences in the trace element contents of hair samples from various racial–ethnic groups have been reported in the literature. Hung et al. (93) compared the iron : zinc, copper : zinc, and calcium : zinc ratios in scalp hair from 20 Vietnamese students with those from an equal number of their Polish counterparts. Both groups lived under identical conditions in a student hostel in Krakow. The iron : zinc ratio of the former group was approximately half that of the latter, and the calcium : zinc ratio of the former was half again greater than that of the latter. The copper : zinc ratios for both groups were the same. When presented as the ratios to sulfur, the values for copper and zinc were the same in both groups, the iron value for the Vietnamese group was 58% of that for the Polish group, and the calcium value of the former was 155% that of the latter. A significant difference ($p < .002$) was reported between the hair copper levels of whites and blacks from the Lusaka area of Zambia (57). The report, however, did not indicate whether the whites and the blacks lived under identical conditions. Others (60, 93, 95) have compared differences in trace element concentrations of the hair from various racial–ethnic groups, but the reported differences may be due to either geographical or environmental factors.

There is controversy in the literature as to whether or not the trace element levels in scalp hair from males differs from those of females. Some investigators have reported significant differences between the sexes; others have found no such differences. Some representative data for copper, iron, and zinc are presented in Table 2.2.

Reeves et al. (90) found the mean lead concentrations in scalp hair from males did not differ significantly from that of females at the 90% confidence level. Klevay (96), however, reported that the lead content of hair from females was significantly higher than that from males. Chattopadhyay et al. (8) have observed the opposite; that is, the hair of males showed consistently higher levels of lead than the hair of females of the same age group and from the same habitat.

In other reports, mean hair calcium and magnesium concentrations for females were found to be twice the values found for the males (89, 97), and the nickel

Table 2.2 ▪ Concentrations of Copper, Iron, and Zinc in the Hair of Males and Females, mg/kg[a]

	Males		Females		
	Number	Mean ± SD	Number	Mean ± SD	Reference
Iron	37	4.2 ± 3.7	70	4.8 ± 5.0	T-71
	23	128 ± 76	26	293 ± 235	T-72
	72	31 ± 17	59	34 ± 21	T-74
	116	40 ± 28	314	24 ± 11	T-75
	4	53 ± 1.7[a]	2	34 ± 1.5[a]	T-76
Copper	37	18 ± 9.3	70	17 ± 11	T-71
	79	16 ± 1.1	47	56 ± 10	T-73
	97	16 ± 9	93	22 ± 18	T-74
	115	20 ± 12	312	16 ± 17	T-75
	65	13 ± 1.5[a]	65	11 ± 1.3[a]	T-76
Zinc	37	140 ± 61	70	140 ± 77	T-71
	23	195 ± 25	26	221 ± 34	T-72
	82	167 ± 5	47	172 ± 9	T-73
	97	184 ± 66	125	205 ± 93	T-74
	115	115 ± 60	314	80 ± 60	T-75
	65	143 ± 1.2[a]	65	158 ± 1.4[a]	T-76

[a]Geometric means.

T-71. Sakurai, S., J. Iwate Med. Assoc., 1980, 32, 869–884.
T-72. Clemente, G. F., Cigna-Rossi, L., and Santaroni, G. P., in *Nuclear Activation Techniques in the Life Sciences, 1978,* International Atomic Energy Agency, Vienna, 1979, pp. 527–543.
T-73. (62).
T-74. (57).
T-75. Gershoff, S. N., McGandy, R. B., Nondasuta, A., Pisolyabutra, U., and Tantiwongse, P., Amer. J. Clin. Nutr., 1977, 30, 868–872.
T-76. Wiesner, W., Görner, W., Niese, S., Baldauf, K., Grund, W., Hennig, M., and Mende, T., Isotopenpraxis, 1980, 17, 277–282.

contents of female hair were found to exceed those of male hair by a factor of four (62, 98).

Until such time as the contradictions are resolved, careful considerations must be given to the age, race, and gender of the subjects from whom hair samples are collected. Comparisons of trace element concentrations in human scalp hair should be made between age-matched, gender-matched cohorts.

2.4. Hair Color

Hair color is another variable that may be responsible for variations in the trace element concentrations of hair from different subgroups of the population. Hair color is determined by the amount of melanin pigments in the cortex. Dark hair has higher amounts of these pigments than does blond or white hair. Red hair contains, in addition, siderin pigments. The siderin pigments contain iron (99), and the biosynthesis of the melanin pigments involves copper as a cofactor for tyrosinase (100). Hence, there may be a relationship between trace elements and hair color.

As early as 1951, Dutcher and Rothman (101) reported that the iron content of red hair was higher than that of blond or black hair. The iron concentrations were 97.8, 24.3, and 27.1 mg/kg, respectively. No relationships between hair color and hair copper concentrations were observed.

Schroeder and Nason (62) have found that black hair from males had a significantly higher magnesium concentration than did blond, brown, or red hair from males. For females, they found that the magnesium concentration in red hair was greater than that in blond hair. Other differences they observed were (a) for both sexes, blond hair contained less zinc than did black, brown, white, or red hair; (b) for males, red hair had a higher nickel content than did male brown hair; and (c) for males, black hair was lower in cadmium and higher in lead than were the other colors of hair for males. No differences on the basis of color were observed for copper or chromium. Eads and Lambdin (61) have also reported no differences in the copper contents of hair on the basis of hair color. They did, however, observe a significantly higher zinc content in the darker colors of hair of both sexes.

Dorea and Pereira (102) have also evaluated hair zinc and copper concentrations on the basis of hair color in a population of 150 Brazilian boys. Their study may be unique in that, in addition to visually classifying hair color as blond, light brown, dark brown, or black, they established a quantitative color classification based on the spectrophotometric determination of melanin content. From their study, they concluded that "hair color defined and divided into four different ranges of melanin concentration does not affect the concentration of zinc or copper in head hair" (p. 2380).

Although copper is involved in the synthesis of melanin, there appears to be some agreement that the hair color is independent of the concentration of this element in the hair. On the other hand, the zinc content of hair does appear to vary with hair color. In the case of other trace elements, the situation is not at all clear. More information is certainly needed on this aspect of hair trace element levels.

2.5. Geographical Habitat

The levels of the trace elements in the hair of inhabitants of one geographical location appear to differ significantly from the levels in the hair of those residing in a different location. These differences have, in some cases, been attributed to differences in the levels of environmental pollutants from location to location. In other cases, the differences may be due to genetic and/or dietary factors for specific racial–ethnic groups.

Eads and Lambdin (61) have proposed that the hair of residents of Port Arthur, Texas, contained 36% more lead than the hair of residents of Hanover, New Hampshire, because the former were exposed to higher airborne lead concentrations from a gasoline production center at Port Arthur. The sevenfold difference (4.3 versus 27.6 mg/kg) between hair lead concentrations of residents of Los Alamos, New Mexico, and those of Chicago residents may also be due to airborne lead from gasoline (105). Klevay (96) has also noted differences in hair lead concentrations on the basis of a rural–urban gradient and concluded that "only individuals or groups which have been matched for age, sex, and place of residence may be compared" (p. 172) for the assessment of lead exposure by hair analysis. The correlations of hair lead levels with the rural–urban gradient have also been reported by Chattopadhyay *et al.* (8). Airey (38) has evaluated the mercury concentrations in hair of 559 residents from 32 locations in 13 different countries. The mean values for the various subgroups (ranging from 0.5 mg/kg in Ontario, Canada, to 16.7 mg/kg in Lake Murray, New Guinea) were only partially related to fish consumption. Geographical and geological factors may also have been involved.

Industrialization may also play a role in the concentrations of trace elements in hair. Jervis *et al.* (104) found the highest levels of lead in the hair of those residing within 300 m of lead refineries. Similarly, they found the highest arsenic levels in the hair of those residing near a gold refinery. In a study involving over 2000 children from different cities, Baker *et al.* (105) noted that the hair arsenic levels were highest for those living in towns with copper smelters and that the children from towns with zinc smelters had the highest cadmium levels in their hair. Elevated hair arsenic levels have also been reported for the hair of those living in the vicinity of a coal-fired power plant in Czechoslovakia (106) and of those living in industrialized parts of Austria (107). Bhat *et al.* (108) have reported elevated manganese levels in the hair of those residing in the vicinity of a fossil-fuel-based power station.

Qureshi *et al.* (60) have measured the levels of a dozen trace elements in hair samples from 105 Pakistani, and they compared their mean results with those reported for residents of India, Iraq, Japan, the United States, and England. Some of their data are presented in Table 2.3. Arunachalam *et al.* (79) have also reported

Table 2.3 ▪ Trace Element Concentrations in Hair from Residents of Different Countries[a]

Element	Geometric means, mg/kg					
	Pakistan	India	Iraq	Japan	U.S.A.	England
Cu	8.6	15.3	—	11.4	15.0	20.6
Mn	2.9	2.5	—	0.5	0.1	1.3
Zn	245	128	165	179	164	261
Fe	41	50	106	—	30	—
Co	0.2	0.05	0.2	0.04	0.03	—
Cr	1.0	0.3	2.6	—	1.5	—
Au	0.1	—	0.03	0.01	—	0.05
Ag	0.2	0.4	0.4	0.3	—	—
Sb	0.1	0.1	1.2	—	1.7	0.4
As	0.2	0.07	0.3	—	0.1	0.5
Se	1.0	1.3	0.9	0.7	1.2	—
Hg	1.2	—	0.7	3.8	1.8	3.5

[a] After Qureshi et al. (60).

differences in the trace element contents of hair from 260 students residing in various parts of India, and Clemente et al. (109) have similarly reported differences for 49 subjects from five different regions of Italy.

2.6. Use of Dietary Supplements and Medicines

Arunachalam et al. (79) have measured the concentrations of 21 elements in hair samples from 260 subjects. When the results were processed through a pattern-recognition approach, using principal-component analysis and a minimal-spanning tree, they found that the vegetarians and nonvegetarians formed two distinct groups. Hunt et al. (110) found no significant difference between the mean zinc levels in hair from 106 control subjects and that from 107 subjects receiving a daily vitamin and mineral supplement providing 20 mg of zinc. The mean values and standard deviations were 184 ± 41 and 175 ± 38 mg/kg, respectively. Lane et al. (111) were also unable to demonstrate an increase in hair zinc levels after 5 weeks of zinc supplementation, but Greger and Geissler (112) have reported an increase in the zinc concentrations of hair during 95 days of supplementation. The consumption of a highly refined diet, however, may be responsible for reduced hair zinc levels (113). The calcium content of hair also appears to reflect calcium consumption (114).

Oral contraceptives are among the medications reported to affect the concentration of trace elements in hair. Deeming and Weber (115) have reported decreased copper and increased zinc in the hair of those using these agents. Klinger et al. (116) reported increased zinc, decreased silicon and chromium, and no changes in copper, manganese, gold, or cesium in the hair of those using oral contraceptives. Vir and Lowe (117) found that oral contraceptive use had no effect on hair zinc and copper levels. Other pharmaceuticals reported to affect the levels of trace elements in the hair are gold (118) and copper (119), used for chrystotherapy and the treatment of Menkes's syndrome, respectively. Leishmaniasis patients who are treated with N-methylglucamine antimoniate are reported to show elevated concentrations of antimony in their hair (119a).

To avoid possible confusion in the interpretation of hair trace element levels, the dietary habits and medical histories of the donors should be recorded and considered.

3

Assessment of Nutritional Status

Schroeder (120) identified the essential trace elements as those necessary for biological function. Under homeostatic conditions, the intake of essential trace elements equals the output, and the nutritional requirements of the biological system are met. Although these requirements differ from system to system and from element to element, standards have been established or recommended in most cases. In addition to measuring the dietary inputs and excretory outputs, nutritional status has been assessed by measuring the trace element levels in various body tissues and fluids and comparing the results to normal values.

More than 20 years ago, Strain *et al.* (9) proposed the use of scalp hair as a "reliable, simple, and atraumatic method for assessing zinc body stores" (p. 245). Subsequent studies (121) have supported this proposal, but others (122) have raised questions about the relationship of the zinc levels in hair to the levels in other tissues. These questions have been reviewed by Combs *et al.* (123) and by Rivlin (37) for zinc, as well as for other essential trace elements.

3.1. Essential Trace Elements

The list of essential trace elements has more than doubled during the past quarter century. This increase is due, in part, to the sensitivity and selectivity of the modern analytical techniques used for trace element determinations. Trace elements are included in or excluded from the list on the basis of current research. Hence, there are differences of opinion on the status of the same trace elements.

Sanders (124) has chosen to classify the essential trace elements into three groups:

Group I   Those that the human body requires in well-defined amounts
Group II   Those that are needed by the human body, but in what exact amount is not yet determined
Group III   Those that are required by various types of animals, but they have not yet been found to be needed by humans.

He has placed iron, iodine, and zinc in Group I; copper, manganese, cobalt, molybdenum, selenium, and chromium in Group II; and tin, vanadium, fluorine, silicon, nickel, and arsenic in Group III. Faulkner (125) does not include arsenic in his listing of essential trace elements, but he does include calcium, phosphorus, chlorine, potassium, sulfur, sodium, and magnesium in a secondary listing of major elements in the human body. Olwin (126) has identified chromium, cobalt, copper, fluorine, iodine, iron, manganese, molybdenum, nickel, selenium, silicon, tin, vanadium, zinc, and possibly arsenic as essential trace elements on the basis of current evidence, with the proviso that "all of the information is not in" (p. 247). Some of the functions of the essential trace elements are presented in Table 3.1.

3.2. Manifestations of Mineral Deficiencies

Among the factors that may produce the clinical symptoms of essential trace element malnutrition are

1. Inadequate dietary intake
2. Impaired intestinal absorption
3. Poor bioavailability
4. Excessive excretion
5. Antagonisms with other elements.

Chromium is in Sanders's Group II. Schwartz and Mertz (127) reported that a low-chromium status in rats and monkeys was associated with impaired glucose

Table 3.1 ▪ Some Biochemical Functions of the Essential Trace Elements in Humans and/or Animals

Element	Function
Chromium	Required for glucose metabolism
Cobalt	Component of vitamin B_{12}
Copper	Component of oxidative enzymes, required for hemoglobin synthesis
Fluorine	Essential for normal growth in rats
Iodine	Component of thyroid hormones
Iron	Component of hemoglobin; component of oxidative enzymes
Manganese	Component of enzymes
Molybdenum	Component of oxidative enzymes
Nickel	Essential for normal growth in rats
Selenium	Component of oxidative enzymes
Silicon	Needed for normal growth in rats
Tin	May function in oxidation–reduction catalysis
Vanadium	May function in oxidation–reduction catalysis
Zinc	Component of enzymes

metabolism. Chromium supplementation was subsequently shown to improve impaired glucose tolerance in some diabetics, geriatric subjects, and malnourished children, but not in others. "Chromium is only one of the many factors possibly related to the increase of diabetes and diseases related to it" (p. 128). In addition to impaired glucose tolerance, chromium deficiency has been associated with retarded growth, decreased glycogen reserves, increased incidence of aortic lesions, and disturbances in amino acid utilization for protein synthesis (14).

Cobalt, which is also in Sanders's Group II, is perhaps unique in being essential to humans only in the form of vitamin B_{12}. The tissues of human and nonruminant animals cannot synthesize vitamin B_{12}. Deficiencies of this vitamin result in pernicious anemia, retarded growth, glossitis, and spinal-cord degeneration.

Although copper was identified as an essential trace element more than 50 years ago (129), it carries a Sanders's Group II classification. Copper serves an important function as a component of oxidative enzymes such as tyrosinase, cytochrome oxidase, and monoamine oxidase. A deficiency of copper can result in depressed white-cell levels, impaired bone formation, and anemia. The anemia stems from the involvement of copper in mobilizing iron for hemoglobin formation. Copper deficiency causes a depigmentation of the hair, probably resulting from depressed tyrosinase activity in the conversion of tyrosine to melanin.

Fluorine, which is in Sanders's Group III, has been identified as a potentially essential trace element for growth and development in rats (130). Messer *et al.* have reported that low-fluoride diets result in decreased hematocrits (131) and decreased fertility (132) in rats. While not necessarily related to nutritional status, the positive effects of fluoride supplementation on dental health are well documented (133).

Sanders has classified iodine as a Group I trace element. Iodine was identified as essential to the human body more than 125 years ago (134). The recommended daily allowances (RDAs) of iodine are 40–50 μg for infants, 70–120 μg for children, and 150 μg for adults. For pregnant and lactating adults, the RDAs are 175 and 200 μg, respectively (135). Iodine deficiency often results in simple goiter, the compensatory enlargement of the thyroid. If this compensation does not provide sufficient iodine trapping and tri- and tetraiodothyronine-synthesizing capacity, the metabolic rate of the body is reduced. Extended iodine deficiency causes retarded physical development and mental capacity in the young. In adults, the result is myxedema, a milder manifestation of cretinism.

Iron is also classified as a Group I element by Sanders. MacMunn (136) identified iron as an essential trace element 100 years ago. For infants and children, the RDA is 10–15 mg. Nonpregnant adults should receive 10–18 mg, and the RDA for pregnant adults is 30–60 mg (135). Anemia is a frequent consequence of iron deficiency. Severe iron deficiency is also associated with an increase in serum triglyceride concentration (137, 138), which may be related to a reduction in lecithin-cholesterol acyltransferase (139).

There is little doubt about the essentiality of manganese, but the body's requirement for this element has not yet been established. Sanders has, therefore, classified it in Group II. Fifty years ago, Kemmerer *et al.* (140) demonstrated a relationship between manganese deprivation and growth retardation in mice. Forty years later, Doisy (141) reported that manganese deprivation in an adult human male resulted in weight loss, transient dermatitis, nausea, retarded growth of nails and facial and scalp hair, and hypocholesterolemia. The addition of manganese to the diet reversed these abnormalities. Dietary manganese intake ranges from 0.5 to 12.5 mg per day (142), and the absolute daily requirement has been estimated as 1.0 mg (143).

Molybdenum is in Sanders's Group II. Although Underwood (144) has not identified a significant role for molybdenum in human and animal nutrition, others (145, 146) have found that it is a catalytically essential prosthetic group in several enzyme systems. Molybdenum deprivation has been reported to cause deficiencies in sulfite oxidase and xanthene oxidase, which are reversed by supplementation (147). The daily molybdenum requirement for humans has been estimated as from 100 to 200 μg (148).

Nickel, a Sanders's Group III element, is essential for normal development of chicks and rats (149, 150). Nickel activates numerous enzyme systems, some of which are crucial in human and animal metabolism (151). Evidence for nickel deficiency in humans has not been found, and recommendations for the human daily requirement of nickel have not been made.

Selenium is in Sanders's Group II. It was identified as a toxic trace element prior to being recognized as an essential micronutrient. Selenium deficiency has been related to Keshan disease, a cardiomyopathy endemic in a region of China in which the major food crops are grown in soil of very low selenium content (152). This selenium-deficient region and the epidemiologic characteristics of Keshan disease have been described by Iyengar and Gopal-Ayengar (152a).

Selenium deficiency also results in suppression of glutathione peroxidase activity, but the suppression is reversed with selenium supplementation (153). While the RDA for selenium has not been firmly established, from 50 to 200 μg has been estimated as a safe and adequate daily intake (122).

Silicon is also in Sanders's Group III. Chicks (154) and rats (155) fed silicon-deficient diets show depressed growth. The silicon appears to be involved in the formation of bone and connective tissue. Human silicon deficiency has not been demonstrated, and an RDA for silicon has not been established.

Although the biological function of tin is not defined, it appears to be necessary for normal growth in the rat (156). The Sanders's classification for tin is Group III, and the dietary intake for normal nutrition is estimated as from 4 to 16 mg (157).

Like the other elements in Sanders's Group III, vanadium deficiency has resulted in retarded growth and development in chicks (158) and rats (159). Deficiency states have not been reported in the human, nor has the basis for vanadium essentiality been determined.

Zinc has been known as an essential trace element for more than 50 years (160). It has a Group I Sanders classification. Zinc is a cofactor for more than 200 enzyme catalyzing processes for the following: nucleic acid and protein synthesis, cell division, tissue growth, cellular immunity, epithelial integrity and wound healing, sexual maturation and function, neuropsychological function, and the senses of taste, smell, and vision (152). The manifestations of zinc deficiency in the human, which are reversed by zinc supplementation, include stunted growth, hypogonadism, roughened skin, and impaired sense of taste. For infants, the zinc RDA is 3.5 mg. Children should receive 10 mg of zinc daily, and the RDA for adults is 15 mg. Pregnant and lactating adults should receive 20 and 25 mg, respectively (135).

3.3. Applications in Human and Animal Nutrition

Passwater and Cranton (27) have published extensive discussions on (1) how mineral nutrients and elemental pollutants affect human health, and (2) how the determination of trace elements in human scalp hair may identify deficiencies of essential trace elements and exposures to toxic elements. The utilization of hair analysis for these purposes remains, however, the object of much conflict and controversy.

The work of Strain et al. (9) is among the first applications of hair analysis to the assessment of zinc status. As mentioned in an earlier chapter, they report a mean zinc concentration of 54 ± 5.5 ppm in the hair of Egyptian dwarfs with demonstrated zinc deficiencies, compared to a value of 103 ± 4.4 ppm for the hair of normal Egyptians. Oral zinc sulfate therapy produced a mean zinc level of 121 ± 4.8 ppm and clinical alleviation of the zinc deficiency syndrome in the dwarfs. Hambidge and his co-workers (163) have correlated zinc levels of less than 70 ppm in the hair of Denver children who showed some of the symptoms of zinc malnutrition: poor appetite, retarded growth, and hypogeusia. After 1-3 months of daily dietary supplementation with 1-2 mg zinc per kg of body weight, taste acuity was restored to normal.

On the other hand, Gershoff et al. (164) were not able to correlate hair levels of zinc (as well as of iron and magnesium) with differences in height, weight, hemoglobin, or morbidity in 430 Thai children generally regarded as retarded in growth and development. McKenzie (165) concluded from her study of 110 adult New Zealanders that the measurement of zinc in serum, urine, hair, and/or toenails does not provide a sensitive indication of the nutritional status with respect to this element. Gibson and DeWolfe (166) found no evidence for intrauterine malnutrition on the basis of zinc, copper, and vanadium concentrations in hair from low-birth-weight, full-term infants and from preterm infants. The hair from the preterm infants did, however, contain less iodine and vanadium than did the hair from the control and low-birth-weight, full-term infants. Subsequently, Gibson (167) proposed that the decline in hair zinc levels during the first 12 neonatal months suggested suboptimal zinc status. She attributed this to inadequate zinc intake. Dorea et al. (168, 169) found no relationship between low zinc levels in hair and malnutrition, but the malnutrition was not identified as zinc deficiency. Earlier, however, Dorea (170) reported quite the reverse: "a significantly higher zinc concentration in hair of normal children compared to the malnourished group" (p. 2324). Hunt et al. (110) found a decline in the hair zinc levels of pregnant adults who received a zinc supplement to their slightly deficient diets. The serum zinc levels, however, responded positively during the course of the treatment. One of the conclusions from this study was that hair zinc concentrations were not significantly correlated with dietary zinc intake. Kohrs *et al.* (171) reported that pregnant subjects who did not drink alcohol had higher hair zinc concentrations than those who did drink alcohol.

The literature abounds with contradictions about the relationship between hair zinc levels and the dietary zinc conditions. Lines and Bell (172), for example, reported that hair zinc levels were below normal for children with suspected zinc deficiency. Ren *et al.* (173) similarly found that the zinc levels in hair from underdeveloped adolescents were distinctly lower than those from well-developed adolescents in China. On the other hand, Erten *et al.* (174) reported that the zinc levels in the hair of malnourished children were significantly higher than those from their healthy, age-matched cohorts. O'Leary *et al.* (175) also proposed a negative correlation between hair zinc levels and growth parameters on the basis of their work with 6-month- to 4-year-old children from a low-income region of rural Costa Rica. The opposite relationship, a positive correlation between scalp hair zinc levels and the height and weight of children under 2 years of age, was reported by Gentile *et al.* (176). A positive correlation between hair zinc levels and height and weight was also reported by Heinersdorff and Taylor (177) on the basis of their study of 219 English school children in the 10- to 11-year-old age group. Bradfield *et al.* (178), however, have presented data indicating no difference in hair zinc and copper levels for normal and malnourished Peruvian children. Vivoli *et al.* (179) have also reported that "the distribution of zinc and copper in serum and hair related to auxological situation have not shown any significant differences among the auxological groups investigated" (p. 512) in a study involving 542 Italian students aged 11 to 13 years.

McDonald *et al.* (180) and Higashi *et al.* (181) have observed no significant differences in the zinc or copper concentrations in hair from infants who were breast-fed and in hair from infants who were fed formulas containing lesser amounts of these elements. In a subsequent study, however, Matsuda *et al.* (182) reported that the zinc levels in infant hair were increased in response to feedings with a zinc-enriched formula.

Hair zinc levels were also increased in response to zinc acetate supplement in adults suffering zinc deficiency due to uremia (183). Taste acuity and sexual function were also improved by this supplement. It is the positive reports that cause Gupta *et al.* (184) and Chen and Ren (185) to support the use of hair zinc levels for the assessment of zinc nutrition. But it is the inconsistencies such as the foregoing that lead to the publication of articles entitled "Hair Analysis: Worthless for Vitamins, Limited for Minerals" (186), "Misuse of Hair Analysis for Nutritional Assessment" (37), and "Commercial Hair Analysis: Science or Scam?" (186a).

Hair analysis has also been utilized to investigate human nutritional status with respect to metals other than zinc. Klevay (46) reported that the copper contents of hair samples from more than 200 Panamanian subjects varied with both age and gender. A positive correlation, demonstrated more strongly for postpuberty females than for preadolescents, between scalp hair copper levels and blood serum copper concentrations was found. Klevay (46) concluded that only age-matched, gender-matched cohorts could be used in comparing copper nutriture on the basis of copper concentrations in scalp hair. Neither Vir and Lowe (117) nor Gibson (187) found correlations between the copper concentrations in hair and those in serum, and Bradfield *et al.* (188) reported that hair copper levels remained normal when there was clear evidence for copper deficiency in the diet. Panday *et al.* (189) have shown that serum copper level, as well as the levels of zinc, calcium, and magnesium in serum from malnourished Indian children, were lower than those of matched controls.

Izumi (114) has reported that hair calcium levels paralleled dietary calcium intake. Machida *et al.* (190), however, found that the addition of calcium to the diet of calcium-deficient rats resulted in a decrease in hair calcium levels.

Izumi (114) also reported a possible relationship between the iron content of hair and the iron content of the diet. Herber *et al.* (191) have also reported that the iron content of the hair was positively related to the daily dietary intake of iron.

Yang *et al.* (192) have proposed that Keshan disease resulted from selenium deficiency and was characterized by depressed selenium levels in the hair. Gallagher *et al.* (193) have found hair analysis to be a valuable tool for assessing selenium status. They found dietary supplementation with selenium-enriched yeast was reflected by significant increases in hair selenium levels. While the supplementation resulted in increased hair levels, it was not reflected in whole-blood selenium levels, and there was no correlation between the hair and blood concentrations of selenium. Earlier, Xiashu *et al.* (194) found a significant correlation between the scalp hair levels and the blood plasma levels of selenium when the diets of Keshan disease victims were supplemented with inorganic selenium.

Clemente *et al.* (195, 196) compared the dietary intake of antimony, cesium, chromium, cobalt, iron, mercury, rubidium, selenium, silver, and zinc with the corresponding concentrations of these elements in urine, feces, blood, and hair for four population groups in Italy. Intake and excretion, with the exception of cesium, did not differ greatly among the groups. Good agreement with literature values was observed for cobalt, iron, rubidium, selenium, and zinc. The hair concentrations of cobalt, chromium, nickel, and zinc from two of the population groups were found to be higher than those of the others. The blood levels did not show corresponding differences. It was concluded that external sources, rather than dietary intake, were responsible for the elevated levels of these elements in the hair.

The determination of trace elements in hair has also been applied to assessing the nutritional status of livestock. This application has recently been reviewed by Combs *et al.* (123) and by Kulachenko (197). Some specific applications are listed in Table 3.2.

The assessment of nutritional status on the basis of hair trace element levels appears to have been more successful for livestock than it has been for humans. This may be due to a higher degree of environmental and nutritional homogeneity among the animal species. Nonetheless, there are serious differences of opinion on the

Table 3.2 ■ Applications of Hair Analysis to Assessing the Nutritional Status of Livestock

Reference	Elements	Animals	Asessment of nutritional status
T-77	Ca, Cu, Fe, Mg, Mn, P	Pigs	Hair contents were of limited value for assessing nutritional status
T-78	Ca, Co, Cu, Fe, K, Mg, Mn, Zn	Dairy cows	Hair contents reflected pasture grass composition
T-79	Ca, Cu, Fe, K, Mg, Mn, Mo, Na, P, Se, Zn	Beef cattle	Hair contents reflected pasture grass composition
T-80	Ca, P	Dairy cows	Hair contents reflected diet
T-81	As, Ba, Br, Cd, Ce, Co, Cr, Cs, Fe, K, La, Na, Pb, Sb, Sc, Se, Sm, Th, Zn	Cows	As, Ba, Ce, Fe, La, Se, Sm in hair correlated with pasture, other elements were poorly correlated with contents of pasture
T-82	Co	Calves	Hair is only suitable indicator of cobalt reserves in the body
T-83	Co, Cu, Mn, Zn	Cows	Dietary supplementation increased levels in milk but not in hair
T-84	Cu	Pigs	Hair content did not reflect marasmus-like or kwashiorkor-like diets
T-85	Cu	Sheep	Hair contents reflected wet-season dietary deficiency
T-86	Cu	Horses	Hair contents were poorly correlated with soil contents
T-87	Cu	Calves	Hair content reflected dietary supplement
T-88	Cu	Calves	Hair content reflected dietary supplement
T-89	Cu	Bulls	Hair content reflected dietary supplement
T-90	Cu, Fe, Mn	Cattle	Hair contents reflected Cu and Mn deficiencies
T-91	Cu, Mn, Zn	Cattle	Hair contents correlated with clinical symptoms of deficiency and levels in alfalfa and soils
T-92	Cu, Zn	Cattle	Hair contents reflected Cu and Zn deficiencies
T-93	Cu, Mn, Mo, Zn	Cows	Hair contents reflected Cu and Mn deficiencies
T-94	Li	Goats	Hair content correlated with clinical symptoms of deficiency, depressed levels in organs and tissues, and dietary intake
T-95	Mg, P	Cattle	Hair Mg contents correlated with levels in forage and in organs and tissues in the wet season

(*continued*)

Table 3.2 ▪ (*Continued*)

Reference	Elements	Animals	Asessment of nutritional status
T-96	Mn	Cows, pigs	Hair content reflected dietary levels, hair content not correlated with levels in other tissues and organs
T-97	Mn	Goats	Hair content did not reflect dietary supplement, hair content correlated with liver content
T-98	Mn	Cattle	Hair content was of no value for assessing nutritional status
T-99	Mo	Goats	Hair content reflected dietary deficiency, hair content correlated with levels in other tissues and organs
T-100	Mo	Horses	Hair content reflected dietary excess
T-101	Na	Cows	Hair content did not reflect dietary supplement
T-102	S, N	Calves	Hair and blood S and N increased in response to dietary S increase
T-103	Se	Cows	Hair content correlated with concentrations in blood and pasture grass
T-104	Se	Horses	Hair content did not reflect pasture level
T-105	Se	Cows	Hair content reflected dietary intake
T-106	Zn	Cattle	Hair content did not reflect dietary supplement

T-77. Kornegay, E. T., Thomas, H. R., and Bartlett, H. S., J. Anim. Sci., 1981, 52, 1060–1069.
T-78. Bondareva, N. I., Dokl. Tskha., 1976, 200, 80–85.
T-79. Szabo, F., Allattenyesz. Takarmanyozas, 1982, 31, 53–60.
T-80. Peteva-Vancheva, Z., and Ilieva, I., Zhivotnovud. Nauki, 1977, 14, 3–9.
T-81. Ronneau, C., and Cara, J., Sci. Total Environ., 1984, 39, 135–142.
T-82. Pythoun, J., Plickova, V., Stolc, L., Miskovsky, Z., and Zagick, F., Zivocisnd. Vgroba, 1979, 24, 413–420.
T-83. Bakan, V. N., Ovsishcher, B. R., Bondareva, N. I., and Alimzhanov, B. O., Izv. Timiryazeusk. S-kh. Akad., 1978, 3, 173–178.
T-84. Bradfield, R. B., and Pond, W., Amer. J. Clin. Nutr., 1980, 33, 2224–2225.
T-85. Gyang, E. O., Ogunbiyi, O., and Hull, M., Bull. Anim. Health Prod. Afr., 1981, 29, 107–109.
T-86. Hatak, J., Sb. Provozne Ekon. Fak. Ceskyck. Budejovicich Vys. Sk. Zemed. Proze. Biol. Rada, 1977, 15, 83–94.
T-87. Istomina, N. L., Nauchn. Tr. Leningr. S-kh. Inst., 1978, 353, 71–78.
T-88. Judson, J. G., Dewey, D. W., McFarland, J. D., and Riley, M. J., Bull. Environ. Contam. Toxicol., 1974, 11, 626–630.
T-89. Regius, A., Szuss, E., Szollosi, I., and Weber, A., Z. Tierphysiol. Tierernaehr. Futtermittelkd., 1982, 47, 169–175.
T-90. Majewski, T., Krupinski, A., Bialkowski, Z., and Zabek, S., Med. Weter., 1978, 34, 558–559.
T-91. Nazarov, S., Rish, M. A., and Shukurova, D. E., Nauk. im. V. I. Lenina, 1982, 7, 32–34.

(*continued*)

Table 3.2 ▪ (*Continued*)

T-92.	Abdullaeu, D. V., Mukumov, K. R., and Rish, M. A., Tr. Biogeokhim. Lab. Akad. Nauk. SSSR, 1976, 14, 130–154.
T-93.	Anke, M., in *13th International Conference Proceedings on the Grasslands*, E. Wojahn and H. Thoens, eds., Akad. Verlag, Berlin, 1980, pp. 1477–1479.
T-94.	Anke, M., Gruen, M., Groppel, B., and Kronemann, H., in *The Biological Importance of Lithium*, Mengen-Spurenelem, Arbeitstag, M. Anke and H-J. Schneider, eds., Karl Marx University, Leipzig, 1981, pp. 217–239.
T-95.	Kistoko, M., McDowell, L. R., Bertrand, J. E., Chapman, H. L., Pate, F. M., Martin, F. G., and Conrad, J. H., J. Anim. Sci., 1982, 55, 28–37.
T-96.	Kovalski, V. V., Vorotnitskaya, I. E., and Fartelberg, R. U., Tr. Biogeokhim. Lab. Akad. Nauk. SSSR, 1980, 18, 155–161.
T-97.	Koyama, T., Miyamoto, S., and Takahashi, T., Chikusan Shikenjo Kenkyu Hokoku, 1983, 40, 31–38.
T-98.	Mehnert, E., Arch. Exper. Vet. Med., 1984, 38, 16–20.
T-99.	Anke, M., Kronemann, H., Hoffmann, G., Gruen, M., and Groppel, B., Mengen-Spurenelem, Arbeitstag, M. Anke and H-J. Schneider, eds., Karl Marx University, Leipzig, 1981, pp. 211–216.
T-100.	Cape, L., and Hintz, H. F., Amer. J. Vet. Res., 1982, 43, 1132–1136.
T-101.	Wegner, T. N., and Schuh, J. D., J. Dairy Sci., 1983, 66, 924–926.
T-102.	Boshyan, G. M., and Kuzmina, E. V., Tr. Vses. Nauchno. Issled Inst. Vet. Sanit., 1976, 55, 36–41.
T-103.	Ishida, N., Suski, H., and Kawashima, R., Nippon Chikusan Gakkai Ho, 1983, 54, 275–279.
T-104.	Ogura, Y., Ushimi, C., and Urehara, N., Nippon Chikusan Gakkai Ho, 1981, 52, 823–824.
T-105.	Ogura, Y., and Ushimi, C., Norin Suisansho Kachiku Eisei Shikenjo Kenkyu Hokoku, 1981, 82, 41–45.
T-106.	Beeson, W. M., Perry, T. W., and Zurcher, T. D., J. Anim. Sci., 1977, 45, 160–165.

usefulness of assessing nutritional status based on the trace element concentrations of scalp hair. Critics of hair analysis, in some cases, confused general malnutrition with specific mineral deficiencies. Consequently, the lack of significant correlations between the levels of zinc, copper, and other specific trace elements in hair from malnourished subjects and that from the normal population is to be expected. In addition, the critics have assumed that blood levels of essential trace elements are directly related to nutritional status. If this is not the case, the failures to demonstrate correlations between blood and hair levels of trace elements is also to be expected. On the other hand, in many cases, the proponents of hair analysis have not shown quantitative relationships between trace element levels in hair and their metabolic activities. Reilly (113), for example, maintains that "hair analysis remains a useful, noninvasive procedure for monitoring dietary intake of metals under defined circumstances" (p. 143), but she does not define the circumstances. Clearly, more research is needed to fully define the relationships between the levels of essential trace elements in scalp hair and the nutritional status of the hair donor. At present, the research is incomplete, and the assessment of nutritional status on the basis of trace elements in human scalp hair is premature.

4

Identification of Systemic Intoxication

The use of hair analysis to identify systemic intoxication has been popularized by Weider and Hapgood (198). They have written a historical detective story, *The Murder of Napoleon,* based upon both Forshufvud's initial research (2, 3) and contemporary documentation from the memoirs of those actually present at Longwood House on St. Helena from 1815 to 1821. The authors present Forshufvud as a toxicologist–detective who discovered one of history's greatest crimes 150 years after it was committed.

Historically, the interests of the toxicologist have been directed toward the physiological effects of heavy metals. Cadmium, mercury, and lead were recognized as occupational hazards long ago, and compounds of arsenic and thallium have been used as commercial poisons for many years. These elements have no known biological function, and their presence in the biological system often interferes with the normal biological processes. According to Bowen (199), "All elements, including the essential ones, are toxic at high concentrations" (pp. 129–130). He cites the use of copper sulfate as an algicide to make his point, and he presents the idealized growth response curves for essential and nonessential elements to demonstrate the difference between essentiality and toxicity. These curves are presented in Figure 4.1. Selenium has a very narrow optimum range: It is both an essential and a toxic element. The essential–toxic assignment for arsenic is not yet clear.

4.1. The Toxic Elements

Cadmium was recognized as an occupational hazard a century ago, on the basis of its acute toxicity. The chronic toxicity of cadmium became known in 1955 as the painful consequences of bone decalcification in postmenopausal victims of *itai itai byo*. In the 15 years that followed, 200 cases of this disease, half of which resulted in death, were recorded in the Jintsu River Valley. The disease was caused by the

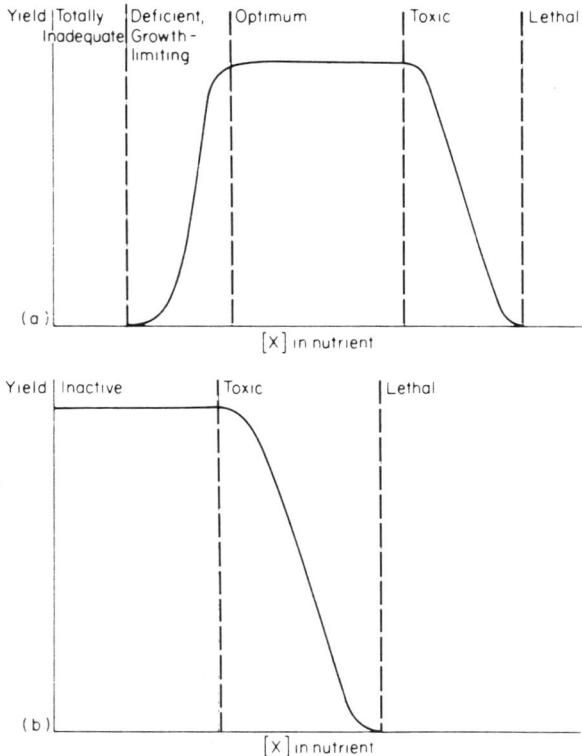

Figure 4.1 • Idealized diagrams showing the yield of an organism as a function of the concentration of an element X in the nutrient supplied. (a) X essential: (b) X nonessential.

ingestion of food and water contaminated with cadmium, and it was characterized by (a) rheumatic symptoms with intense pain in the joints, resulting from the loss of bone materials, and (b) the bones becoming as flexible as soft tissue (200).

Cadmium ingestion also resulted in damage to the kidneys: renal tubular dysfunction. Some epidemiological evidence appears to relate cadmium accumulation with hypertension. The mechanisms of cadmium toxicity are ill defined at present. They may involve inactivation of sulfhydryl-containing enzymes, competition with zinc, and inhibition of copper absorption.

The toxicology of mercury parallels that of cadmium. The acute toxicity of mercury was identified in the workplace long before its chronic toxicity to the general public was suspected. Beginning in 1953, increasing numbers of adults and children residing near Minamata Bay showed loss of coordination, numbness of the limbs, partial blindness, and loss of hearing. Convulsions, coma, and death followed in 46 of 125 cases. By 1956, "congenital Minamata disease" was observed in the offspring of symptom-free parents. The disease was subsequently diagnosed as acute methyl mercury poisoning and traced to the consumption of fish that had concentrated, biomagnified, mercury from industrial wastes discharged into Minamata Bay (201).

The toxicity of mercury involves both tissue destruction and enzyme inactivation. Gastroenteritis, nephritis, and hepatitis are frequent consequences of mercury poisoning. Mercury poisoning also causes irreversible neurological damage. Circulatory or central nervous system (CNS) collapse is often the cause of death from mercury poisoning (202).

Until recently, the domestic use of leaded gasoline released approximately 1 kg of lead for every man, woman, and child in the United States each year. Even though the United States has required lead-free automotive fuels for more than a decade, lead poisoning from a variety of domestic and industrial sources remains a subject of concern because its effects on the nervous systems of children given to pica and on fetuses and newborns of mothers ingesting lead are so severely and permanently damaging (203). The major toxic effects of lead include anemia, renal impairment, and neurological dysfunction (204).

Some of the toxic effects of other elements are summarized in Table 4.1.

4.2. Clinical Observations

Heavy metal poisoning demonstrates classical symptoms and deviations from normal physiology and biochemistry. Because every individual is biologically unique, not every victim of heavy metal poisoning displays all of the symptoms and deviations to the same extent. Hence, a complete medical history supplemented with work records and personal information must be considered, along with these characteristic symptoms.

4.2.1. Mercury Poisoning

Acute poisoning caused by mercury vapor and many mercury compounds is characterized by inflammation of the exposed mucous membranes. Hence, stomatogingivitis, pneumonitis with respiratory distress, cough, fever, abdominal pain, vomiting, and diarrhea are typical symptoms. Permanent renal damage may be a result. Constriction of the visual fields, ataxia, and difficulty with speech are typical signs. Death may result from hemorrhage and either circulatory collapse or renal tubular necrosis.

Limited exposure to organomercurials often results in fatigue, memory loss, and poor concentration ability. Chronic exposure to inorganic mercury can lead to weakness, weight loss, anorexia, tremor, and uncontrolled mood swings, ranging from depression, shyness, nervousness, and irritability to irrational temper outbursts.

The laboratory diagnosis and assessment of chronic mercury poisoning is frequently aided by urinalysis. Urinary excretion, preferably over a 24-hour period, is a good index of mercury exposure. Normal output is less than 0.05 μmol/L (205).

Table 4.1 ▪ Some Consequences of Elemental Intoxication

Element	Toxic effects
Aluminum	Chronic inhalation of aluminum dusts may produce pulmonary damage, fibrosis of the lungs, encephalopathy, and bronchopneumonia
Antimony	Acute poisoning may result in vertigo, abdominal cramps, nausea, vomiting, rhinitis, bronchitis, and pneumonitis; liver and kidney degeneration may appear as later signs
Arsenic	Intoxication often results in necrosis of the liver, hepatitis, encephalitis, myelitis, and nephritis, as well as nerve and kidney degeneration
Beryllium	Chronic inhalation often produces weight loss, bone and joint pain, chills, fever, disturbed liver and spleen function, skin lesions, and general physical deterioration
Cadmium	Intoxication produces weight loss, bleeding, rhinopharyngitis, perivascular and peribronchial fibrosis, pulmonary emphysema, and damage to the liver and kidneys
Chromium	Lung and skin cancers are produced by hexavalent compounds; intoxication causes kidney and liver damage
Copper	Acute toxicity may produce nausea, diarrhea, salivation, gastrointestinal hemorrhage, and nephritis
Iron	Chronic inhalation of the oxides may produce a benign pneumoconiosis
Lead	Intoxication causes damage to the CNS and the brain, the reproductive system, and the kidneys
Manganese	Chronic inhalation may cause headache, insomnia, apathy, pneumonitis, and bronchitis
Mercury	Damage to the liver, kidneys, brain, and CNS result from intoxication
Selenium	Intoxication may result in kidney and liver damage, as well as damage to the CNS and brain
Thallium	Intoxication causes gastrointestinal hemorrhaging, peripheral neuritis, necrosis of the liver, delirium, and coma; death is usually due to CNS or circulatory collapse
Zinc	Acute toxicity may cause diarrhea, lassitude, and tremors

4.2.2. Lead Poisoning

Sweet metallic taste, salivation, vomiting, intestinal colic, and lowered body temperature are symptoms of acute lead poisoning. There may also be cerebral edema, convulsions, and coma. Kidney damage is frequent, and peripheral neuropathy often causes wrist drop. The cause of death is usually cardiovascular collapse.

Chronic lead poisoning has CNS manifestations. These are most pronounced in children, and they include irritability, headache, insomnia, restlessness, and ataxia. Later, confusion, delirium, convulsions, and coma may develop. Muscle paralysis involving the extensor muscle of the wrist and foot may result from neurologic degeneration at the horn cells of the spinal cord.

The gastrointestinal symptoms of chronic lead poisoning result from stimulating the smooth muscle of the gut. They often include distension after meals, constipation, nausea, vomiting, and colic. Appetite loss, weight loss, and fatigue usually follow. A black or purple line sometimes forms at the margin of the gums when lead in the saliva is precipitated with sulfide produced by gingival bacteria. Arsenic, bismuth, mercury, and tin produce similar precipitates at the gingival border.

Hematologic characteristics of chronic lead poisoning are basophilic stippling and elevated lead content. Urinary lead concentration is also elevated, as are the urinary coproporphyrins (206).

Campbell and Baird (207) have reported on the symptoms and treatment of lead poisoning in a group of demolition workers. Many of the workers were found to have blood lead levels in excess of 3.8 µmol/L, which was the upper limit for the industrially exposed population in the United Kingdom (U.K.). Urinary coproporphyrin excretion exceeded the normal 500 nmol/24 hours. Weakness or tiredness, anemia, abdominal pain, blue line (probably the aforementioned black or purple line), nausea and vomiting, pleuritic pain, constipation, and elevated blood urea were observed in most of the cases. Other clinical features were anorexia, headache, hyperuricemia, metallic taste, joint pain, peripheral neuropathy, irritability, and insomnia.

4.2.3. Arsenic Poisoning

The symptoms of acute arsenic poisoning usually begin a half hour after exposure and include a tightness in the throat and stomach pain. Vomiting and intense diarrhea quickly follow. The output of urine is characteristically depressed. Death from total collapse usually results within a few days, but death that occurs up to 14 days after acute arsenic poisoning is caused by nephritis.

In chronic arsenic poisoning, diarrhea and vomiting occur, but these are less pronounced than they are in cases of acute arsenic poisoning. Tremors and peripheral neuritis are present in some cases. The afferent motor and sensory nerves in the lower extremities are affected. Ankle jerk disappears, and leg muscles atrophy.

Arsenic stimulates the horny layers of the skin, which leads to the appearance of dark brown scales. Skin keratoses frequently result from prolonged exposure to arsenic, and these may become malignant.

4.3. Relationships between Toxic Elements in Hair and Their Concentrations in Fluids and Other Tissues

In order to assess heavy metal poisoning, it is necessary to identify the dispositions of the toxicants. Information of their distributions and excretions as well as the dependencies of these processes on time and dosage is required. While it is possible to obtain such information from human victims of accidental or deliberate poisonings, animal experiments are superior for reasons of experimental design, experimental control, and experimental reproducibility.

Gregus and Klaassen (208) have reported a study on fecal, urinary, and biliary excretion and the tissue distribution of 18 metals in male rats after intravenous administration. The metals studied were arsenic, bismuth, cadmium, cesium, chromium, cobalt, copper, gold, iron, lead, manganese, methyl mercury, mercury, selenium, silver, thallium, tin, and zinc. Their distributions into liver, kidneys, spleen, heart, lung, pancreas, intestine, stomach, testes, muscle, bone, brain, blood, and plasma were evaluated after 1, 2, 3, and 4 days at four different doses of each metal. One of the results of this study was "it demonstrates that disposition of various metals is vastly different" (p. 37).

4.3.1. Cadmium Dispositions in Animals

Animal experiments have been employed to study the relationships between the concentrations of cadmium in hair and in other tissues. Kollmer and Berg (209) found that the distributions of cadmium in liver, kidney, blood, brain, and hair were proportional to dose for up to 3 months after intravenous administration, and that the uptake and excretion of cadmium appeared to depend upon liver–blood–kidney relationships. No direct relationship between cadmium deposited in hair and any one of the other tissues could be demonstrated. Subsequently, Kollmer (210) demonstrated that the deposition of cadmium in rat hair was dependent upon the growth stage of the hair as well as upon the blood cadmium concentration from intravenous injection. Kollmer (211) then demonstrated that cadmium administered to the rat by gastric intubation was deposited in the hair in amounts dependent upon the dose and independent of the amounts of cadmium accumulated in other tissues from prior exposures.

Wesenberg *et al.* (212) found significant correlations between the cadmium dose and the cadmium content of teeth, hair, blood, kidney, liver, spleen, heart, muscle, and adrenal gland after 10 weeks of graded dosings in drinking water, using the rat as his experimental model for chronic exposure. Wesenberg (213) later used interrupted dosings to simulate acute exposures and found significant correlations between the cadmium contents of the indicator organs (blood, hair, and teeth) and the target organs (kidney, liver, spleen, heart, muscle, and adrenal glands). From this latter study, he also found that cadmium passed the placental and mammary barriers, and that deposition was increased by the presence of lead. Still later, Wesenberg (214) reported that chronic cadmium exposure affected copper and zinc metabolism in the rat to a lesser extent than did acute cadmium exposure.

The aforementioned works of Kollmer and Wesenberg indicate that there are relationships between hair cadmium concentrations and the concentrations of cadmium in organs such as the liver and kidneys. Others, however, have reported contrary findings. Machida *et al.* (190) have reported that the liver and kidney cadmium concentrations increased, and the bone and hair cadmium concentrations remained unchanged, in rats receiving 10 subcutaneous injections of cadmium chloride over a 15-month period.

Weigel *et al.* (215) conducted a study on cadmium accumulation in rats after 60 days of dietary exposure to cadmium oxide. They found, relative to controls, no increase in the cadmium concentrations of the hair, bone, blood, and testes, but the liver, lung, kidney, and spleen showed significantly elevated cadmium concentrations. Some of the inconsistency may be due to the differences in the administrations of the cadmium compounds. Intravenous injection is certainly not the same as subcutaneous injection, and the administration of soluble cadmium in drinking water may not be equivalent to feeding rats a synthetic casein diet supplemented with cadmium oxide.

4.3.2. Mercury Deposition in Animals

Ohmori and Hashimoto (216) have reported on the tissue distributions of mercury in guinea pigs after a 6-month chronic exposure. Mercury doses corresponding to 0.27, 2.7, and 27 ppm were added to the diet for 25 weeks, and the animals were then fed a mercury-free diet for the next 8 weeks. The control animals received the mercury-free diet throughout the 33-week period. Hair samples were collected during the 33-week period. The animals were sacrificed at the end of this period, and the mercury contents of the tissues were determined by radiochemical neutron activation analysis (NAA). Relative to the controls, the tissues from the exposed guinea pigs showed dose-related mercury levels. For the animals receiving 27 ppm mercury in the diet, kidney mercury levels were elevated more than 100 times normal, and the liver mercury levels were elevated to almost 50 times normal. Most of the other tissues, including the hair, from the exposed animals had mercury contents approximately 10 times larger than those of the controls.

Berg and Kollmer (40) previously have shown elevated mercury levels in the hair of rats exposed to mercury by either intravenous injection or by gastric intubation. The guinea pig may be a superior animal model for such studies because its random hair-growth patterns more closely approximate the growth of hair on the human scalp. Scheiner et al. (217), however, were unable to demonstrate an elevation in the nickel concentrations of hair from guinea pigs whose drinking water was fortified with 2.5 ppm nickel for 4 months.

4.3.3. Indications from Animal Studies

On the basis of the aforementioned controlled animal experiments, it appears that exposure to cadmium and mercury is reflected by elevated levels of these elements in the internal organs and in the hair. There also appears to be a dose-related response. Yokel (218) has reported dose-dependent increases in the hair and peripheral organ aluminum concentrations for rabbits receiving five subcutaneous injections of aluminum lactate weekly for 4 weeks. Jacob et al. (47) found firm correlations between dietary copper supplement, 3.2 ppm, and the copper concentrations in the hair and liver of rats.

4.4. Applications to the Recognition of Acute and Chronic Poisoning in Humans

Accidental and deliberate poisonings of human beings with heavy metals have occurred in the consumer, domestic, and occupational environments. In many of these instances, accurate histories of the clinical symptoms have been correlated with the concentrations of the heavy metals in hair and other tissues from the victims.

4.4.1. Arsenic Poisoning of Humans

Chronic arsenic poisoning has been caused by arsenic-contaminated drinking water. Hindmarsh *et al.* (219) reported one such instance in Waverly, Nova Scotia. They examined 92 residents of Waverly after two cases of arsenic poisoning led to the discovery of 29 contaminated wells in the town. Of these, 27 had clinical features that could be attributed to chronic arsenic poisoning. A positive relationship was established between the frequency of these symptoms and the concentrations of arsenic in the hair and in the drinking water of the victims. Valentine *et al.* (44) were able to show that the arsenic concentrations of blood, urine, and hair were correlated with the arsenic concentrations of the drinking water in two California and four Nevada communities. Olguín *et al.* (220) correlated the arsenic concentration of drinking water from the Comarca Lagunera region of Mexico with the arsenic concentrations in the blood, urine, hair, and nails for residents with the cutaneous signs of arsenic poisoning and for those with known arsenic exposures. In the Valentine *et al.* and the Olguín *et al.* studies, the hair arsenic concentrations appeared to show a dose response. Relationships between the clinical symptoms of arsenic poisoning and the concentrations of arsenic in hair and/or drinking water have also been made in Chile (221) and in the Hungarian Peoples' Republic (222, 223). Similar relationships have been established for chronic poisoning from airborne arsenic associated with the combustion of coal in Czechoslovakia (224), the smelting of copper in the United States (225), and the general urban atmosphere in the People's Republic of China (226).

Yamamura and Yamauchi (227) have investigated the possibility of arsenic poisoning in the occupational environment. While they found that the arsenic levels in the urine, blood, and hair of workers exposed to As_2O_3 dust were significantly higher than those of the control group, no relationship with clinical symptoms was possible: both groups were asymptomatic. On the other hand, Feldman *et al.* (228) were able to relate peripheral neuropathy to the arsenic concentrations of hair and urine of workers in a copper smelter, who were occupationally exposed to As_2O_3. Gabor *et al.* (229) also found elevated levels of arsenic in the hair and urine of smelter workers. These elevated levels were correlated with high rates of dyspepsia, astereovegetative, and polyarthralgic symptoms.

Pirl *et al.* (230) describe the case of a 9-year-old boy who died of unknown causes. He had been hospitalized twice for gastrointestinal distress, muscle fatigue, and various neurological dysfunctions. He recovered and was discharged into the care of his family. Two weeks before his death, he was again hospitalized for similar symptomatology and again improved rapidly in the hospital environment. Suddenly, his condition worsened, and he expired within 24 hours. It was later established that his mother had brought some milk to him in the hospital on the previous day. The arsenic content of his hair was found to be 16 ppm at the proximal end and approximately 0.1 ppm at the distal end.

The Murder of Napoleon was mentioned in the beginning of this chapter. It is possible that the 9-year-old described by Pirl (230) and Napoleon were indeed victims of deliberate arsenic poisoning. Leslie and Smith (231) have subsequently confirmed that the distribution pattern of arsenic in hair taken from Napoleon in 1816 was similar to that observed after the daily ingestion of excessive amounts of arsenic. Lewin and his co-workers (232) have analyzed a different, but authentic, sample of Napoleon's hair and found its arsenic content to be normal. Grodzins (233) has evaluated three samples of Napoleon's hair. Each was certified to have been cut from Napoleon's head at the time of his death. Two of the samples showed no evidence of arsenic. This inconsistency is more likely due to a faulty authentication process than to questionable laboratory results. The chronic exposure to arsenic is reflected by elevated hair levels of this element.

4.4.2. Lead Poisoning in Humans

Chronic lead poisoning has resulted from the continued use of lead-containing consumer products, the long-term ingestion and/or inhalation of lead compounds in the domestic environment, and the exposure to lead and its compounds in the workplace. In many instances, the characteristics of chronic lead poisoning include elevated levels of lead in the hair, as well as in the other tissues.

Kopito and his colleagues (43, 234) have firmly identified relationships between the concentration of lead in the hair of children and the major clinical and laboratory findings associated with chronic plumbism in children. The mean lead level of hair from children with lead intoxication was 10 times greater than that of the controls (i.e., 282 versus 24 ppm). The source of the lead in most cases was attributed to pica. Marzulli and Maibach (234a) established a correlation between blood-lead and hair-lead levels in children identified in a lead-poisoning surveillance project. From linear regression, they found the following:

$$\text{Whole blood lead} = 39.79 + 0.02757 \times \text{Hair lead}$$

when the whole blood lead concentration is expressed as micrograms per 100 milliliters, and the hair lead is expressed as milligrams per kilogram (the correlation coefficient was $r = .854$; for the 11 blood–hair data points, $p < .001$).

Niculescu *et al.* (235) investigated the relationships between blood-lead and hair-lead levels in two groups of adults with different occupational exposures to airborne lead. Group 1 consisted of 31 subjects exposed to high concentrations of lead in the air. Of these, 26 had blood-lead concentrations in excess of 40 μg/dl. Group 2 consisted of 33 subjects with low exposures to airborne lead. Of these, 28 had blood-lead concentrations below 40 μg/dl. The hair-lead levels were evaluated with respect to age of the subject, hair color, and blood-lead level. The only significant correlation was between hair-lead level and blood-lead level for the subjects in Group 1 (the correlation coefficient $r = .72$, and $p < .001$). Clayton and Wooller (236) have measured the blood-lead and hair-lead levels of 38 male workers from a lead–acid battery factory. The blood-lead–hair-lead correlation was significant ($r = .76$, and $p < .0005$). The data were fitted to an exponential curve of the following form:

$$\text{Hair lead} = 15.2 \ e^{(0.067 \ \times \ \text{Blood lead})}$$

where the hair-lead concentration is expressed in micrograms per gram and the blood-lead concentration is expressed in micrograms per 100 milliliters.

4.4.3. Mercury Poisoning in Humans

Chronic mercury poisoning has resulted from the continued use of consumer products containing this toxic element, as well as from the ingestion, inhalation, and/or absorption of mercury from food, air, and water in the domestic and occupational environments. Elevated mercury levels in hair and other tissues often accompany chronic mercury poisoning.

The suspected chronic systemic mercury intoxication of six women, from the long-term use of skin bleach creams containing ammoniated mercury, was reported by Marzulli and Brown (54). Mercury etiology was confirmed in one of these cases, where the skin bleach was used for more than 4 years and the concentrations of mercury in urine, blood, and hair were 250 μg/24 hours, 100 ng/ml, and 125 mg/kg, respectively. In the other cases, the symptoms were attributed to other causes (i.e., psychosomatic, carpal tunnel syndrome, and peripheral neuropathy of unknown cause).

Sherlock *et al.* (237) maintain that "except for occupationally exposed individuals, consumption of fish is the main source of exposure of man to mercury" (p. 271). In their study of fish consumption by almost 1000 persons living in either one or the other of two coastal regions of the United Kingdom (U.K.), they found a well-defined relationship between mercury in blood and mercury in hair when exposure is prolonged and relatively constant. The straight line fitted to their data is as follows:

$$\text{Hair mercury} = 0.367 \times \text{Blood mercury} + 0.694$$

where the hair mercury concentration is expressed in milligrams per kilogram, and the blood mercury is expressed in micrograms per liter. Matthews (238) has also reported elevated levels of mercury in blood and hair as a result of consuming fish contaminated with mercury. Hansen, Wulf, and Kromann (41) investigated the possibility of chronic systemic intoxication by mercury in a population of Greenlanders who consumed mercury-contaminated seal. They found a correlation between hair and blood mercury concentrations (i.e., $r = .9222$). Their relationship was demonstrated by the following equation:

$$\text{Hair mercury} = 289 \times \text{Blood mercury} + 63.4$$

where the hair mercury concentration is expressed in micrograms per kilogram and the blood mercury is expressed in micrograms per liter. The slope of 289 agrees with the value of 367, when reported by Sherlock et al. (237), when the hair mercury concentration for the latter is expressed as micrograms per kilogram. Such agreement is indicative of a firm relationship between the mercury concentrations of hair and the mercury concentrations of blood.

4.4.4. Thallium Poisoning in Humans

Thallium, on a weight-for-weight basis, is more toxic than lead. One of the clinical features of thallium poisoning is hair loss. Typical symptoms of chronic thallium poisoning are sleep disorders, headache, fatigue, and gastrointestinal dysfunctions.

Brockhaus et al. (239) identified a population of thallium-poisoned individuals living in the vicinity of a cement plant that emitted a thallium-containing dust. Relative to two control populations, those living near the cement plant showed elevated thallium in both urine and hair, but no positive correlation could be established between the hair-thallium concentrations and urinary-thallium concentrations, hair loss, skin alterations, or gastrointestinal dysfunctions. Kijewski (240) found elevated levels of thallium in the hair, blood, and urine after attempted suicides. He was also unable to establish positive correlations. On the basis of their studies of hair collected from medical students who were poisoned with thallium, Metter and Vock (241) concluded that thallium caused trophic disorders in keratin formation, and the resulting structural alteration led to alopecia. That thallium has such a marked effect on hair metabolism may be the reason for the lack of a correlation between the levels of thallium in the hair and in other tissues and fluids.

5

Diagnosis of Diseases

The absence of a specific essential trace element from the diet usually results in specific signs of nutritional deficiency, and the ingestion of an excess of a toxic element usually produces characteristic symptoms of heavy-metal poisoning. The exact role of trace elements in human illness–wellness, however, is much more complex than their essentiality or toxicity. The trace elements are often involved in the activity of enzyme systems. More than 90 zinc enzymes have been identified to date (242), and there are almost an equal number of copper enzymes (243). Abnormal metabolism—disease—may involve enzymes different from those active during normal metabolism—health. These differences may result in changes in the trace element composition of the metabolic milieu from which the hair is formed. In this respect, specific changes in the trace element composition of the hair may reflect deviations from normal metabolism. It is frequently not possible to speculate on whether the trace elements are the cause or the result of the disease.

Correlations between the trace element concentrations in hair and specific diseased states, other than those associated with dietary deficiency or systemic intoxication, have been identified. Some of these correlations have been independently summarized in various review papers (20, 21, 72, 244). They include a correlation between cystic fibrosis and both elevated sodium and depressed calcium concentrations in hair, as well as a correlation between hypoglycemia and both elevated calcium and depressed potassium concentrations in hair.

5.1. Role of Trace Elements in Disease

Hemochromatosis or hematosiderosis is attributed to an increase in iron absorption. Typical manifestations are cirrhosis of the liver, a peculiar bronze pigmentation of the skin, diabetes mellitus in over half of the victims, and various kinds of cardiomyopathy. Pituitary failure is not uncommon. Abdominal pain, arthritis, and chondrocalcinosis occur less frequently. These changes are all thought to result from parenchymal iron deposition.

Acrodermatitis enteropathica is a lethal, autosomal, recessive trait, which usually occurs in infants of Italian, Armenian, or Iranian lineage. The manifestations of the disease include progressive bullous-pustular dermatitis of the body orifices and extremities, combined with paronychia and generalized alopecia. Ophthalmic signs may include blepharitis, photophobia, conjunctivitis, and corneal opacities. Severe gastrointestinal disturbances (chronic diarrhea, malabsorption, steatorrhea, and lactose intolerance) and neuropsychiatric disorders (emotional disorders, irritability, tremor, and occasional cerebellar ataxia) are symptomatic of acrodermatitis enteropathica. Cachexia, usually with terminal respiratory infection, is usually the cause of death. The disease is ultimately traceable to the malabsorption of zinc due to abnormalities of Paneth's cells in the intestinal mucosa. The abnormalities may be of genetic origin.

Menkes's kinky hair syndrome is a sex-linked abnormality caused in infants by a defect in the intestinal absorption of copper. The affected infants show depressed copper and ceruloplasmin that lead to progressive cerebral degeneration, retarded growth, abnormally sparse and brittle hair, arterial lesions, and scurvy-like bone changes.

Wilson's disease is inherited as an autosomal recessive trait, and it occurs most frequently in the children of consanguineous marriages. The result is the progressive accumulation of copper in various body tissues: erythrocytes, kidney, liver, and brain. Copper absorption appears to be accelerated. Asymptomatic hepatic copper accumulation begins early in the course of the disease. After the fifth year or so, the copper-binding capacity of the liver becomes saturated, and excess copper is released. The uptake of excess copper by the erythrocytes causes an acute hemolytic anemia. Hepatic insufficiency may develop, and this results in a hepatocellular necrosis for 30–50% of the victims. The hepatic manifestations may resolve, or they may produce cirrhosis with ascites, edema, and progressive hepatic failure. The neurologic syndrome begins when the cerebral copper accumulation is sufficient to destroy nerve cells. The common neurologic features are tremor of one or both of the upper extremities, choreoathetoid movements, rigidity of the skeletal muscles, dysarthria, and personality changes leading to dementia. Wilson's disease also leads to renal complications.

Ritland and Aaseth (245) have surveyed liver cirrhosis with respect to excess iron from hemochromatosis and to excess copper from Wilson's disease. They also identify a reduced level of selenium and a corresponding reduction in the activity of glutathione peroxidase in alcoholic cirrhosis of the liver, and they note that alcoholic cirrhosis of the liver is also accompanied by depressed zinc levels.

Delves (69) has identified the following changes in trace element concentrations as clinically important in identifying some pathological conditions:

Depressed serum copper	Wilson's disease, Menkes's syndrome
Elevated serum copper	Neoplasias, cirrhosis
Elevated urinary copper	Wilson's disease, nephrotic syndrome

Depressed serum zinc	Acrodermatitis enteropathica, neoplasias, cirrhosis
Depressed urinary zinc	Leukemia
Elevated urinary zinc	Cirrhosis, rheumatoid arthritis

The need for accurate and precise determinations of trace elements in defining their specific roles in disease was stressed by Cornelis and Versieck (246). In their review on the subject, they summarized some observed deviations and their possible clinical significance. They reported that the copper, manganese, and zinc contents of serum and packed erythrocytes were changed from their normal values during acute hepatitis, chronic hepatitis, and posthepatitic cirrhosis. They also reported that diseases of the liver and biliary system were associated with changes in the serum molybdenum content. Similarly, uremia was associated with changes in the blood levels of arsenic, bromine, copper, gold, iron, molybdenum, selenium, and zinc, and endemic nephropathy was associated with changes in the blood levels of cadmium, chromium, iron, rubidium, selenium, and zinc. They also cited work in which various cancers were associated with changes in the blood levels of aluminum, calcium, chromium, cobalt, copper, iron, magnesium, manganese, rubidium, selenium, and zinc. They conclude with work on blood rubidium and selenium levels in children suffering from phenylketonuria and maple-syrup-urine disease.

The involvement of trace elements in some diseases is well established. In other cases, unexplained correlations, both positive and negative, have been reported for various diseases and the trace element concentrations of various tissues and fluids. Hair is one of the tissues frequently used to assess the trace-element–disease relationships.

5.2. Correlations of Disease with Hair Trace Element Levels

5.2.1. Cystic Fibrosis

The standard quantitative pilocarpine iontophoresis sweat test is the most reliable single laboratory finding in diagnosing cystic fibrosis. In the newborn, the sodium and chloride concentrations are elevated to values greater than 60 mEq/L. The normal values for neonates are typically below 50 mEq/L.

Kopito et al. (247) reported, "hair of neonates with cystic fibrosis contains significantly elevated concentrations of sodium and potassium" (p. 624). They also reported gross changes in the water solubility or extractability of calcium and magnesium from the hair of cystic fibrosis victims relative to the controls. With respect to the hair samples from the former, nearly all of the calcium and 80% of the magnesium was removed with water, but only small fractions of these elements in the hair samples from the healthy infants were water soluble. The inability of the hair of cystic fibrosis victims to bind calcium and magnesium was identified as the basic defect in this disease.

5.2.2. Hypoglycemia

The aforementioned pilocarpine iontophoresis sweat test remains the standard laboratory procedure for screening and diagnosing cystic fibrosis even though determination of the sodium, potassium, calcium, and magnesium concentrations in the hair was recommended for these purposes 15 years ago. More recently, Stebbing *et al.* (248) have made a connection between hair magnesium and hypoglycemia. They found that reactive hypoglycemic humans had depressed levels of magnesium in hair and blood relative to age- and gender-matched controls. After 6 weeks of magnesium supplementation (340 mg/day) in a double-blind study, the treated group showed normal glucose tolerance tests, and general well-being was improved. One of the conclusions from this work was that reactive hypoglycemia appeared to be a disease of disturbed magnesium balance. Rudolph (249), however, had earlier identified an increase in the calcium: potassium ratio of the hair as characteristic of hypoglycemia.

5.2.3. Reactions to Copper and Nickel

Although Wilson's disease involves copper accumulation, the hair of three male patients with this type of hepatolenticular degeneration was found to contain normal copper concentrations (250). The malabsorption of copper associated with Menkes's kinky hair syndrome can be reversed by copper supplementation (251), but the consequent increases in hair copper concentrations have not been reported (252, 253). Apparently, these diseases are not reflected by corresponding increases or decreases of the hair copper concentrations. Similarly, nickel allergy is not reflected by hair nickel concentrations. Two independent studies (98, 254) have failed to demonstrate significant differences between the concentration of nickel in hair samples from subjects with known hypersensitivity to this element and those from the control populations.

5.2.4. Diabetes Mellitus

Mertz (255) maintains that a meaningful tissue must be selected in order to obtain useful information from trace element analysis. By "meaningful tissue," he means one that is functionally linked to the disease process under investigation, and he goes on to use the diabetes–pancreas link as an example. Ten years after Schwartz and Mertz (127) identified the chromium-containing glucose-tolerance factor, Hambidge *et al.* (15) demonstrated that there was a significantly lower chromium concentration in the hair of children with diabetes mellitus than there was in the hair of their normal counterparts. The geometric mean for the 19 samples from the diabetic children was 0.56 ppm and that from the 33 controls was 0.85 ppm. Hambidge and Rodgerson (256) also reported a significant depression of hair chromium levels in parous women relative to nulliparous controls. Benjanuvatra and Bennion (16) reported that the chromium concentrations in the hair of adult diabetics were significantly lower than those of the nondiabetic controls. The mean values were 0.094 and 0.24 ppm, respectively. These values are approximately four times lower than the aforementioned values for diabetic children and their controls. The children in the Hambidge *et al.* study were residents of the Denver area, and they had a mean age of 7 years whereas all of the subjects in the adult study were Thai, and their mean age was 43 years. The differences between the values from the adult study and those from the study using the children could be due to age, race, and/or habitat. Rosson *et al.* (257) measured the hair chromium concentrations of age-matched, gender-matched groups of insulin-treated diabetics and controls. They found that the mean of the hair chromium concentration of the female diabetic was depressed relative to the female controls, but that of the male diabetics did not differ significantly from the mean of their controls. Rabinowitz *et al.* (258) compared the chromium status of normal men to that of several subgroups of diabetic men. The diabetic men were segregated into obese–nonobese and ketosis-prone–non-ketosis-prone subgroups. The hair and erythrocyte chromium concentrations did not differ significantly among the groups. It appears that the relationship between hair chromium concentrations and diabetes is not as well established as that between chromium and the glucose tolerance factor (259).

5.2.5. Cancer

Cancer is among the adverse effects attributed to excessive exposures to some chromium compounds as well as to compounds of arsenic, beryllium, and nickel. More than a quarter-century ago, Addink and Frank (260) reported on scalp hair zinc levels and cancers, and Lin *et al.* (261) subsequently studied the concentrations of zinc as well as those of copper and iron in hair from patients with esophageal cancer. The latter research group reported that the zinc concentrations in hair and esophageal tissue from patients with cancer of the esophagus were lower than the concentrations of zinc in hair and esophageal tissue from patients with other forms of cancer and from healthy controls. More recent work from the People's Republic of China (262) has also reported that the hair from patients with esophageal cancer shows depressed zinc concentrations, although the concentrations of copper and iron in the hair appear to be elevated by this disease. Scalp hair from Chinese patients with nasopharyngeal carcinomas were found to contain much less copper and zinc when compared to hair from healthy controls (262a). Wiesener and his research group (263) found hair zinc concentrations were elevated in cases of breast cancer, thyroid cancer, and malignant melanoma type of skin cancer. Wiesener *et al.* (264) later reported that the zinc as well as the copper concentrations of cancerous breast tissues were higher than uninvolved neighboring breast tissue. The corresponding geometric means for zinc were 31.4 versus 5.3 ppm. For copper, they were 2.3 versus 0.9 ppm. The scalp hair from those with the mammary carcinoma showed elevated levels of zinc and copper relative to the control population. Typical data are presented in Table 5.1. Mende *et al.* (265) have reported that hair iodine levels are lowered in most diseases of the thyroid; but in cases of cancer

Table 5.1 ■ Effect of Carcinoma on Hair Zinc and Copper[a]

	Control	Mammary carcinoma	Cervical carcinoma
Zinc	148 ± 42	204 ± 47	185 ± 64
Copper	12.2 ± 4.1	15.6 ± 5.4	—

[a]After Wiesener et al. (264).

of the thyroid, the hair iodine levels are increased. Kwiatek et al. (265a) reported that cluster analysis of data for potassium, calcium, manganese, iron, copper, zinc, selenium, bromine, and rubidium concentrations in the hair of patients with cancer of the colon did not differ significantly from those of control subjects. The hair of leukemia patients, however, was found to contain elevated levels of mercury (265b). Thimaya and Ganapathy (266) reported that the concentrations of selenium in both blood and hair tended to be decreased in cancer patients, and that there were no firm correlations between the blood and hair selenium concentrations of the same individual. Moo and Pillay (95) compared the trace element profiles of scalp hair from cancer patients with those of healthy controls and found that iodine was elevated and selenium was depressed. They also reported, contrary to the aforementioned Wiesener finding, depressed zinc concentrations in the hair of cancer patients. These apparent inconsistencies may result from the failure of some investigators to differentiate among the various types of cancers.

5.2.6. Nonspecified Diseases

The failure to carefully specify clinical states renders a comparison of trace element contents of hair from normal and diseased subjects useless. One such report (267) presented data showing elevated chlorine and depressed chromium concentrations in the hair of diseased infants, *but no diseases were identified.* The samples were collected from healthy newborns at the Tokyo Welfare Pension Hospital and from "diseased infants who received some treatment at the same hospital (for example, Muco Cataneous Lymphnode Syndrome = MCLS, and Acuto Hepatitis)" (p. 144). The results were evaluated statistically, and significant differences were reported on the basis of age and gender, but "no characteristic distribution pattern of elements could be found on the individual data of diseased infants" (p. 145). Such comparisons must be made on a disease-by-disease basis. Lacking such information, the data on the concentrations of trace elements in the hair from normal and diseased infants is useless for this purpose. When reports such as this appear in the open literature, publications on the use of trace element levels in hair for the diagnosis of disease lose credibility. Editors and reviewers must bear some of the blame for the publication of such mediocrity.

5.2.7. Keshan Disease

Keshan disease, a childhood cardiomyopathy endemic in some regions of the People's Republic of China, has been attributed to a selenium deficiency. Ying *et al.* (268) found that the selenium levels in the hair and urine of children living in an endemic area were lower than those of children living in a nonendemic area. They also reported that the children from the endemic area retained a larger fraction of orally administered selenium than did the control population.

From this, a positive correlation between Keshan disease and selenium deficiency was assumed. Hsu *et al.* (269) also reported a positive correlation between Keshan disease and selenium deficiency on the basis of depressed blood and hair levels of selenium in children from the endemic area. The hair selenium concentrations were less than 0.129 ppm for the samples from the residents of the endemic area, while the values for the residents of the nonendemic area were greater than 0.167 ppm. This was confirmed by Yang *et al.* (270) in a subsequent study of selenium levels in the diets as well as the concentrations of selenium in the hair and blood samples from the respective populations. They reported, "Most of the population hair contents were below 0.12 ppm in affected areas but it mounted above 0.2 ppm in nonaffected areas," and "the population hair contents averaged 0.07 and 0.343 ppm in affected and nonaffected areas respectively" (p. 199). The selenium concentrations in corn and rice crops from the endemic area were 0.01 and 0.02 ppm, respectively.

Jiang *et al.* (271) investigated the involvement of elements other than selenium in Keshan disease and found no correlations between the disease and the molybdenum and copper concentrations in the hair and blood. None of the preceding studies, however, was able to demonstrate significant differences in the selenium concentrations of hair from Keshan disease victims and that from healthy children residing in the same village or town, nor has selenium supplementation been attempted to prevent the disease.

5.2.8. Kaschin–Beck Disease

Kaschin–Beck disease has also been attributed to selenium deficiency. Li *et al.* (272) have used the appropriate controls in their study of this disease. Of 742 children from the Shanxi province, the mean selenium hair concentration of 389 victims of Kaschin–Beck disease was 0.071 ppm. For the remaining 353 normal children, the mean selenium hair concentration was 0.208 ppm. These values agree with the aforementioned results of Yang for children residing within and outside of the regions where Keshan disease was endemic. The report by Li *et al.* also related lower levels of selenium in soil, crops, and water to higher incidences of Kaschin–Beck disease, and it contained data showing elevated calcium, iron, magnesium, and manganese in the hair of the diseased children. Li *et al.* (273) subsequently demonstrated that depressed hair selenium levels were indicative of Kaschin–Beck disease and that the disease could be prevented by oral selenium supplementation.

Hou and Zhu (274) have also related the environmental selenium concentrations to hair and blood selenium concentrations and the prevalence of Kaschin–Beck disease. Their results confirm those of Li *et al.*, and their recommendations include dietary supplementation with both selenium and vitamin E. Wang (275) has made a comprehensive geographical study of the selenium content of hair from Chinese children with respect to the demography–epidemiology of Kaschin–Beck disease and of Keshan disease. The hair selenium concentrations demonstrated a trimodal distribution: below 0.11 ppm, 0.11 to 0.52 ppm, and greater than 0.52 ppm. The first group resided in regions with low levels of environmental selenium and high incidence of Kaschin–Beck disease and Keshan disease, and the last group resided in industrialized regions and in regions of Northwestern China with high levels of environmental selenium. Yang *et al.* (276) has investigated the environmental selenium levels in Enshi Hubei with respect to the 1961–1964 outbreak of selenium poisoning and found that the soil selenium concentrations were from 25 to 125 times higher in this region than in other regions of China: 7.87 versus 0.059–0.318 ppm.

5.2.9. Myocardial Infarction

Bacso, in many collaborations, has established a relationship between the concentrations of calcium in the hair and the incidence of myocardial infarctions. In 1978, Bacso *et al.* (277) reported that the hair calcium levels of those having suffered myocardial infarctions were significantly lower than those of healthy subjects. The mean values were 910 and 2410 ppm, respectively. Bacso *et al.* (278) later suggested that the determination of hair calcium concentrations could be used to screen the general population for those at risk with respect to myocardial infarction. The recommended warning level was a hair calcium concentration below 700 ppm. Bacso *et al.* (279) developed a procedure for the removal of exogenous calcium from the hair so that the state of health could be better assessed on the basis of the amount of endogenous calcium in the hair. Bacso (280) has also presented data for the calcium concentrations of scalp and facial hair collected from a single individual over a 7-year period. During this time, the hair calcium concentrations for this individual were found to range from a low of 450 ppm to a high of 2200 ppm. It was noted that this range was nearly the same as the ranges observed for groups of individuals, and it was proposed that the causes of these wide variations may be related to the causes for ischemic heart disease. In investigating the postmortem calcium concentrations in hair and the aorta, Bacso *et al.* (281) found that aortic calcium concentrations appeared to increase with increasing gravity of atherosclerosis, and that low hair calcium concentrations showed a slight, negative correlation with aortic calcium concentrations. On the basis of similarities in the lognormal distributions of scalp hair calcium levels, Bacso *et al.* (282) proposed that "the use of scalp hair as a biopsy tissue may become important in assessing some calcium related functions of the body" (p. 387).

5.2.10. Cardiovascular Ailments

Saltman (283) has reviewed the effects of trace elements, both essential and toxic, on the cardiovascular system. He concluded that "neither deficiencies of essential elements nor the presence of toxic heavy metals are primary causes of hypertension in our population" (p. 823). Whanger (284) had previously reported that no relations were observed between blood or hair cadmium levels and blood pressure for residents of Oregon. Medeiros and Borgman (285), however, found that a weak association existed between hair metal concentrations and blood pressure for South Carolina adolescents. Elevated hair copper concentrations were associated with elevated systolic pressures, whereas elevated hair nickel concentrations were associated with depressed systolic pressures, and elevated hair cadmium concentrations were associated with depressions of both systolic and diastolic pressures. They (286) then reported (a) that lower blood pressures were correlated with increased levels of cadmium, calcium, magnesium, and zinc in the hair and (b) that the consumption of salt tended to elevate the blood pressure.

Medeiros et al. (287) subsequently reported a negative correlation between the ratio of sodium : potassium in the hair of male university students from Mississippi and diastolic pressure. In female students from Mississippi, the systolic pressure was negatively correlated with the concentration of sodium in the hair, the concentration of copper in the hair, and the copper : zinc ratio in the hair. No correlations were established between blood pressure and the concentrations of cadmium, chromium, or lead in the hair of this student population. One year later, Medeiros and Pellum (288) reported a positive correlation between diastolic pressure and concentrations of cadmium and lead in the hair of white female adolescents residing in Mississippi and a negative correlation between systolic pressure and the concentration of lead in the hair from their black counterparts. Chen et al. (289) have concluded that hypertension is caused by a dietary deficiency of cobalt. In light of the connections between cadmium and hypertension cited by Passwater and Cranton (27), more positive correlations between hair cadmium concentrations and hypertension would be expected.

5.2.11. Other Diseases

Elevations and depressions of hair trace element concentrations have been reported for victims of Hodgkin's disease, Parkinson's disease, and several other diseases. Some of these are listed in Table 5.2.

5.2.12. Dialysis Treatments

Hemodialysis has also been reported to be associated with changes in the hair trace element concentrations. Tsukamoto et al. (290) reported that hemodialysis had a greater effect on the aluminum and copper concentrations of the hair than it did on

Table 5.2 ▪ Changes in Hair Trace Element Concentrations in Association with Various Diseased States

Disease	Changes in hair	Reference
Cooley's anemia	Depressed Zn	T-107
Childhood cirrhosis	Depressed Zn	T-108
Biliary cirrhosis	Normal Cu	T-109
Epilepsy	Depressed Mn	T-110
Epilepsy	Elevated Mg; depressed Zn	T-110a
Hodgkin's disease	Depressed Zn	T-111
Leprosy	Elevated Na, K, P; depressed Cu, Fe	T-112
Multiple sclerosis	Elevated V, Se; depressed Cu, I, Mn, S	T-113
Multiple sclerosis	Elevated As, Ba, Sb, Se; depressed Al, Au, Br, Cs, I, Mn, Mo, V, Zn	T-114
Parkinson's disease	Elevated Mn	T-115a
Phenylketonuria	Depressed Zn	T-115b
Phenylketonuria	Depressed Se	T-116
Idiopathic scoliosis	Elevated Cu	T-117
Sickle cell disease	Elevated Pb	T-118
Sickle cell disease	Depressed Zn	T-119

T-107. Mazzotta, D., Guarneri, M., and Fagioli, F., Il Farmaco-Ed. Pr., 1986, 41, 388–403.
T-108. Gupta, B. D., and Nirmal, M., Indian Pedi., 1977, 14, 181–184.
T-109. Epstein, O., Boss, A., Margot, B., Lyon, T., David, B., and Sherlock, S., Amer. J. Clin. Nutr., 1980, 33, 965–967.
T-110. Papavasiliou, P. S., and Aronson, R. B., Neurology, 1979, 29, 1466–1473.
T-110a. Shrestha, K. P. and Oswaldo, A., Sci. Total Environ., 1987, 67, 215–225.
T-111. Caudar, A. O., Babacan, E., Arcasoy, A., Erten, J., and Erten, V., Eur. J. Cancer, 1980, 16, 317–321.
T-112. El-Saaiee, L., Abd-el, H., El-Mahdy, H., and Abd-el, G. S., J. Med., 1983, 14, 117–124.
T-113. Ryan, D. E., Holzbecher, J., and Stuart, C. D., Clin. Chem., 1978, 24, 1996–2000.
T-114. Ward, N. I., and Minski, J., Trace Substances in Environ. Health, 1983, 16, 252–260.
T-115a. Sunyapridakul, L., and Bianchine, J. R., Chiang Mai Med. Bull., 1979, 18, 23–31.
T-115b. Lombeck, I., Kasperck, K., Harbisch, H. D., Becker, K., Schumann, W., Schroeter, W., Feinendegen, I. E., And Bremer, H. J., Eur. J. Pedi., 1978, 128, 213–223.
T-116. Lines, D. R., Bell, E. B., Pybus, J., Proc. Nutr. Soc. New Zealand, 1977, 2, 31–37.
T-117. Pratt, W. B., and Phippin, W. G., Spine, 1980, 5, 230–233.
T-118. Olatunbosun, D., Marris, S., Lichte, F., Kairtyohann, S. R., and Vogt, J. R., Trace Substances in Environ. Health, 1976, 10, 383–388.
T-119. Prasad, A., Gov. Rep. Announc. Index, 1978, 69.

Table 5.3 ▪ Changes in Hair Trace Element Concentrations in Association with Various Mental Disorders

Disorder	Trace element changes	Reference
Behavior disturbance	Elevated Cr, Mo, Pb; depressed Co, V	T-120
Behavioral problems	Elevated Al	T-120a
Learning disability	Elevated Cd, Pb	T-121
Learning disability	Elevated Cd, Mn; depressed Cr, Li	T-122
Learning disability	Elevated Se in females; elevated Se, Cd in males	T-123
Learning disability	Elevated Cd, Cu, Mg, Pb	T-120
Dyslexia	Elevated Al, Cd, Cu, Mg	T-124
Cognitive functioning	Elevated Cd, Pb	T-125
Mental retardation	Normal Cu, Mg, Zn	T-126
Mental retardation	Elevated Pb; depressed Na	T-120
Mental retardation	Depressed Ag; elevated Au, Hg, Sc	T-126a
Senile dementia	Depressed Cr	T-127
Senile dementia	Normal Ca, Cu, Mg, Zn	T-128a
Senile dementia	Elevated Al	T-128b
Down syndrome	Depressed Ca, Cu, Mn	T-129
Manic-depression	Elevated V	T-130

T-120. Rimland, B., and Larson, G. E., J. Learn. Disabil., 1983, 16, 1–7.
T-120a. Moon, C. and Marlow, M., Biol. Trace Element Res., 1986, 11, 5–12.
T-121. Pihl, R. O., and Parks, M., Science, 1977, 198, 204–206.
T-122. Pihl, R. O., Drake, H., and Vrana, F., in *Hair Trace Elements and Human Illness, 2nd. ed.*, A. C. Brown and R. C. Crounse, eds., Prager Publishers, New York, 1980, pp. 128–143.
T-123. Ely, D. L., Mostardi, R. A., Woebkenberg, N., and Worstell, D., Environ. Res., 1981, 25, 325–339.
T-124. Capel, I. D., Pinnock, M. H., Dorrell, H. M., Williams, D. C., and Grant, E. C., Clin. Chem., 1981, 27, 879–881.
T-125. Thatcher, R. W., Lester, L. M., McAlister, R., and Horst, R., Arch. Environ. Health, 1982, 37, 159–166.
T-126. Danford, D. E., Smith, J. C., and Huber, A. M., Amer. J. Clin. Nutr., 1982, 35, 958–967.
T-126a. Bhandari, H. P. S., Lal, G., Sidhu, N. P. S., Mittal, V. K., and Sahota, H. S., J. Radioanal. Nucl. Chem. Letters, 1987, 119, 379–385.
T-127. Vorbecky, J., Hontela, S., Shapcott, D., and Vorbecky, J. S., Nutr. Rep. Internat., 1980, 22, 49–55.
T-128a. Dhore, D., Henkin, R. I., Nelson, N. R., Agarwal, R. P., and Wyatt, R. J., J. Amer. Geriatr. Soc., 1984, 32, 892–985.
T-128b. Akanle, O. A., Spyrou, N. M., Damyanova, A. A., Shaw, D. M., and Ali, L., J. Radioanal. Nucl. Chem., 1987, 113, 405–416.
T-129. Barlow, P. J., Sylvester, P. E., and Dickerson, J. W. T., J. Ment. Defic. Res., 1981, 25, 161–168.
T-130. Naylor, G. J., Smith, A. H. W., Bryce-Smith, D., and Ward, N. L., Biol. Psych., 1984, 19, 759–764.

the concentrations of arsenic, bromine, calcium, magnesium, manganese sulfur, vanadium, and zinc. According to Mahajan *et al.* (291), the concentrations of zinc in serum and hair were depressed in both dialyzed and nondialyzed uremic patients, and the clinical signs of zinc deficiency were alleviated after zinc supplementation in a double-blind study involving 25 patients.

Of the 20 elements they studied (Ag, Al, As, Au, Br, Ca, Cd, Cl, Co, Cu, Fe, I, K, Mg, Mn, Na, Sb, Se, V, and Zn), Tomza and Maenhaut (292) found that, relative to 40 controls, the hair iodine concentration of 19 dialysis patients was increased tenfold, and no significant differences were observed for the other elements. Both DeGroot, *et al.* (293) and Marumo *et al.* (294) have studied the aluminum concentrations in hair and other tissues and fluids of dialysis patients in relation to mental problems (hemodialysis encephalopathy or dialysis dementia) associated with metal intoxication in the course of the treatments.

5.2.13. Mental Disorders

Trace element concentrations in hair have been applied to investigating diseases of the mind as well as those of the body. The investigations range from some broad mental disorders (such as learning disabilities and behavioral disturbances) to specific psychoses (such as those of the manic-depressive). Bland (72) has described the potential importance of hair mineral analysis to the diagnosis of mental dysfunction in general. Some specific applications are summarized in Table 5.3.

5.3. Applications as Diagnostic Aids

The medical community has been slow to accept the trace element concentrations in hair as diagnostic indicators of diseases. It is quite clear that the hair-metal-level–disease relationships must be more firmly established in terms of etiology and application before the diagnostic potential of hair mineral analysis can be fully realized. Hair mineral analysis has, on the other hand, found considerable application in the paramedical community. Learning disorders, emotional disturbances, and nutritional deficiencies have been successfully identified and, in some cases successfully treated, on the basis of hair trace element evaluations.

6

Evaluation of Environmental Exposures

The determination of trace element concentrations in hair has been frequently applied to the evaluation of heavy-metal exposures in the domestic and occupational environments. In these applications, hair has been characterized as a biological dosimeter, a recording filament, or, as so eloquently put by Lenihan (295), a "mirror of the environment" (p. 66). The heavy metal contents of the hair reflect both the exposure dose and the absorbed dose. The former is most often established from ambient air and water monitoring programs (296, 297), and the latter, pursuant to U.S. workplace safety and health standards (298), is determined from the blood or urine concentrations of the heavy metals. While hair analysis may not be able to differentiate between the exogenous and the endogenous depositions of the heavy metals, there is no question that the results reflect exposure to heavy metals. Because of the ease with which samples can be collected, transported, stored, and analyzed, hair analysis is valuable in screening individuals and populations for exposures to heavy metals.

6.1. Occupational Exposures

6.1.1. Dentistry-Related Mercury Exposure

More than 15 years ago, Lenihan et al. (299) reported mercury concentrations in scalp and pubic hair from British dentists and their clinical assistants from two to three times higher than the corresponding values from the office staffs at the dental clinics. The respective geometric means with geometric standard deviations are summarized in Table 6.1. The scalp hair values were interpreted as indicative of exposure doses, and the pubic hair values were assumed to reflect absorbed doses. Ten years later, Lin et al. (300) reported geometric means for scalp hair mercury concentrations of 10.77 ± 4.04 and 3.76 ± 1.33 ppm for 32 Taiwanese dental professionals and 30 normal controls, respectively. The arithmetic means for scalp

Table 6.1 ▪ Mercury Levels in Hair of Workers in the Dental Profession[a]

	Scalp hair (geometric means and SDs)	Pubic hair (geometric means and SDs)
Dentists	10.70 ± 2.4	3.85 ± 1.6
Clinical assistants	9.74 ± 2.9	2.98 ± 2.1
Office staff	3.52 ± 1.8	1.59 ± 2.0

[a]After Lenihan et al. (322).

hair mercury concentrations in Korean dentists and their clinical assistants were 8.57 and 5.79 ppm, respectively, while that for residents of Seoul was 2.57 ppm (301). In Jakarta, the average scalp hair mercury concentration of dentists was five times higher than that of the control population (15.51 vs. 2.80 ppm) (302). With the exception of dentists from central Kentucky (303), it appears that occupational mercury exposure results in elevated hair mercury concentrations. The regular analysis of mercury in hair or urine is recommended for monitoring mercury exposure of dental professionals in Japan (304), Great Britain (305, 306), and Poland (307).

6.1.2. Mining- and Refining-Related Exposure

The scalp hair of workers in mining and refining industries has been used to monitor occupational exposure to heavy metals. The hair and urine of Soviet gold miners was reported to show elevated levels of arsenic, reflecting the high concentrations of this element in the mine atmosphere (308). Similarly, the hair of Japanese zinc miners was reported to show elevated concentrations of zinc, copper, manganese, and mercury (309).

Raghupathy and Sharma (310), however, found that the hair zinc concentrations of Indian zinc miners was close to that of the control population and three times less than that of workers from the nearby zinc smelter. The arithmetic means and standard deviations for the three groups were control population, 412 ± 183 ppm Zn; zinc miners, 312 ± 124 ppm Zn; and zinc smelters, 976 ± 573 ppm Zn. The scalp hair of Polish zinc smelters was reported to contain 40 times more selenium, 20 times more arsenic and cadmium, and 10 times more silver than that of the control group (311, 312). In the United States, nonsideropenic anemia among the workers in a copper refinery, coupled with both airborne copper concentrations of from 0.5 to 1 mg/m^3 in the workplace and elevated hair copper, were interpreted as the hemolytic effect of elevated erythrocyte copper (313). Workers in a Romanian copper refinery had a high incidence of dyspepsia, astereovegetative, and polyarthralgic symptoms, and their mean hair and urinary arsenic concentrations were 31 ± 10 mg/kg and 0.12 ± 0.15 mg/L, respectively (239). Feldman et al. (228)

reported that the neuropathic symptoms in American copper refiners were also correlated with the hair and urinary arsenic concentrations. Ohmori (314) found that antimony, arsenic, and zinc, in addition to lead, were elevated in the hair of lead-processing workers. Jamall and Jaffer (314a) found elevated iron concentrations and normal copper and zinc concentrations in the hair of workers at a Karachi steel mill. On the basis of the normal copper and zinc concentrations and the fraction of iron leached from the hair by EDTA solution, they interpreted their findings as reflecting the body burden of iron.

The occupational hazard to workers in the mining and refining industries is almost always airborne. It appears that exposure to such workplace atmospheres is reflected by elevated concentrations of heavy metals in the workers' hair. In some cases, the symptoms of heavy metal poisoning and/or increased concentrations of heavy metals in the workers' urine accompany exposure to these airborne hazards.

6.1.3. Welding-Related Exposure

Welders are also exposed to airborne heavy metal hazards. Manual arc welding of stainless steel with ESAB OK 67-52 electrodes produces a welding fume of the following composition: 5.9% chromium, 20.0% iron, 17.0% manganese, and 1.9% nickel (315). The insoluble hexavalent chromium compounds in such fumes are believed to be carcinogenic (316). Bergert et al. (317) have reported significantly higher manganese concentrations in the hair and urine of welders exposed to manganese in workplace air, and they recommend urinalysis for manganese to monitor the manganese exposure of welders. Wiesener and Grund (318) reported that the average manganese content of hair from welders was five times higher than that in the hair of the controls, and that the serum manganese concentration of welders did not differ from that of the controls. Grund (319, 320) also reported that the geometric mean manganese content of hair from welders was five times higher than that of the controls (respective values were 7.0 and 1.4 ppm). Wiesener and his research group have reported elevations of both chromium and manganese in the hair of welders relative to controls (263). Subsequently, they reported that the chromium in welders' hair exceeded the control value by a factor of three, and they proposed using hair analysis as a dosimeter of exposure to metals (321).

6.1.4. Cadmium Exposure

Ellis et al. (322, 323) were able to determine kidney and liver cadmium concentrations by *in vivo* neutron-capture gamma-ray spectroscopy. They compared these results to the hair cadmium concentrations on a subject-by-subject basis, and they concluded that "hair cadmium levels are not a good index of body burden of cadmium in the industrially-exposed individual" (322, p. 330). Anke (324) found that the hair of occupationally exposed persons contained 165 times more cadmium than the controls, and that the corresponding increases in blood and urine cadmium were 5- and 18-fold. From this, he concluded that the hair cadmium level was not a good indicator of cadmium in the liver or kidneys, but it did reflect cadmium exposure. Brueckner (325) reported 140-fold increase in the hair cadmium concentration of exposed workers, relative to controls, and Brueckner suggested using the hair cadmium content as an indicator of airborne cadmium exposure.

6.1.5. Nondentistry-Related Occupational Exposure to Mercury

Workers in laboratories, chlorine-production factories, and granaries, as well as those in dental clinics, have been exposed to mercury vapor. Cagnett *et al.* (326) have reported that such exposure resulted in elevated mercury concentrations in the hair, blood, and urine. Wiadrowska and Syrowatka (327) found the range of hair mercury concentrations for occupationally exposed workers was 170 to 231 ppm and that for the general population of Warsaw was 0.25 to 7.59 ppm. The mercury concentrations in the blood, urine, and hair of workers in a Spanish chlorine-production factory with the workplace atmosphere containing from 0.05 to 0.1 μg mercury per m^3 were 6.7 μg/100 ml, 0.15 mg/L, and 44 mg/kg, respectively (328). The urine and hair mercury levels of Czech workers who had treated grain with a mercury-containing fungicide were 25 and 300 times higher, respectively, than the values for controls (329). The good techniques of Soviet laboratory workers were reflected in normal (1.42 ppm) mercury hair levels relative to controls (1.05 ppm) (330).

6.1.6. Lead Exposure

Bencko *et al.* (331) found elevated concentrations of lead in the blood and hair of workers in a Prague battery factory, up to 53 μg/100 ml and over 80 mg/kg, respectively, and they proposed the use of hair analysis for monitoring lead exposure. Fergusson *et al.* (332) reported that the concentration of lead in the hair of New Zealand battery factory workers averaged 363 mg/kg. Burguera *et al.* (333a) found that the mean hair lead content of 53 male gas station workers in Merida City, Venezuela, was significantly greater than that of an equal number of age- and gender-matched controls: 48.7 ± 17.5 versus 17.2 ± 8.1 μg/g. The hair lead content of the gas station workers increased with increasing duration of employment. Weber *et al.* (333) reported that the concentrations of lead in the hair of Mexican pottery workers ranged from 3 to 600 ppm while controls ranged from 1 to 40 ppm. One of their conclusions was "the analysis of hair for heavy or toxic metals such as lead, cadmium, mercury and arsenic holds great promise as an indicator of occupational exposure" (p. 1016). Clayton and Woller (236), Dumitru (334), Grandjean (335), and Niculescu *et al.* (235) have also recommended the assessment of lead in hair as a useful screening test for establishing occupational exposure to this element.

6.1.7. Chromium, Arsenic, and Thallium Exposure

Yamamura and Yamauchi (227) reported that urine, blood, and hair arsenic levels were elevated in workers exposed to As_2O_3 dust, and Ndiokwere (336) reported elevated arsenic levels in the hair of workers who applied an arsenic–chromium–copper solution to wood products for protection against fungus and insects. Bertram *et al.* (375) attributed the increased concentrations of thallium they found in the hair of cement plant workers to the "exogenous dust contamination during cement fabrication." The blood and hair of workers in a Romanian dichromate plant were found to contain 0.135 and 83.6 ppm chromium, respectively, while the control values were 0.055 and 0.33 ppm chromium, respectively (338).

Both factory and office workers at a Turkish tannery were found to have hair and urinary chromium concentrations higher than those of controls (339). These values are summarized in Table 6.2. The hair chromium concentrations of the Romanian and Turkish controls agree within a factor of two. It appears that the office workers at the Turkish tannery were also exposed to chromium. This appears not to be the case in a Polish dry cell battery factory where the manganese content of hair from assembly workers was found to be significantly higher than that from colleagues employed as office staff (340).

6.1.8. Summary

Occupational exposure to heavy metals, in many instances, is reflected by elevated concentrations of these heavy metals in the hair. Frequently, elevated blood and/or urinary concentrations accompany the elevated concentrations in the hair, but this is not always the case. In this respect, hair can be used to monitor heavy metal exposure in the occupational environment, and it can serve as a screening test for heavy-metal systemic intoxication. The latter, however, must be confirmed by more extensive clinical and laboratory evaluations.

6.2. Nonoccupational Exposures

A possible consequence of metal mining and refining is the pollution of the immediate industrial site as well as the contamination of the contiguous environ-

Table 6.2 ▪ Occupational Exposure to Chromium[a]

Exposure	Urine Cr, ng/ml	Hair Cr, mg/kg
Factory worker	6.6 ± 1.2	17.4 ± 3.6
Office worker	2.3 ± 0.5	14.5 ± 2.9
Control	0.2 ± 0.03	0.56 ± 0.07

[a]After Saner *et al.* (339).

ment. Heavy-metal exposure of those residing in such environments has been monitored with hair analysis. Hammer *et al.* (5) clearly demonstrated that the hair of fourth-grade schoolboys residing in cities with lead and zinc smelters contained significantly more cadmium and lead than did the hair of schoolboys residing in cities without smelters. For the five cities studied, the hair concentrations of arsenic, cadmium, and lead reflected the city-to-city exposure dose gradients, while the mean copper and zinc concentrations in hair from each of the five cities were constant. Typical arithmetic means and standard deviations for lead and zinc are listed in Table 6.3.

Jervis, Chatt, and their co-workers have made several studies of pollution from smelters in and around Toronto. Lead levels as high as 20 times normal were reported in the hair of children living close to secondary lead refineries (341). The hair lead concentrations of people residing within 500 m of lead refineries were found to be 10 times those of the control population (104). Median values for the concentrations of lead in hair from rural, urban, and smelter area residents were 9.1, 15.3, and 48.5 ppm, respectively, and a blood-lead–hair-lead correlation was obtained for these subjects (8).

Baker *et al.* (105) studied the chronic exposure of young children living within 6 km of 19 different primary lead, zinc, or copper smelters. Nearly 1800 blood, hair, or urine samples were collected and analyzed for arsenic, lead, and cadmium. The hair arsenic and urinary arsenic concentrations were elevated (2.6 vs. 0.1 mg/kg and 0.019 vs. 0.006 mg/L, respectively) for the children living near the 11 copper smelters. For the children living within 6 kg of the 5 zinc smelters, the hair and blood showed increased cadmium (5.6 vs. 0.9 mg/kg and 0.0036 vs. 0.0020 mg/L, respectively). The concentrations of lead in the hair of the children living near the 3 lead smelters were significantly higher than those of the controls (77 vs. 13 mg/kg), but both groups had blood lead concentrations of 0.16 mg/L. This was interpreted as "indicating substantial external exposure" (p. 267). As might be expected, "consistently negative correlations were found between the distance of a child's residence from the smelter and the level of cadmium, lead, and arsenic in the hair" (p. 265).

Sonneborn (342) also reported that exposure decreased with increasing distance

Table 6.3 ▪ Lead and Zinc Concentrations in Hair of Nonoccupationally Exposed Schoolboys

City	Lead, mg/kg	Zinc, mg/kg
I	107 ± 132	154 ± 34
II	44 ± 49	145 ± 31
III	14 ± 14	156 ± 26
IV	12 ± 11	155 ± 37
V	8 ± 5	154 ± 33

from the smelter. Milosevic *et al.* (343) have reported data for the cadmium and lead concentrations in the hair of subjects living within 5 km of a lead smelter, using age- and gender-matched cohorts living more than 20 km from the smelter as controls. None of the subjects or controls had a history of occupational exposure to heavy metals. Their mean results for males were hair cadmium, 2.7 versus 1.9 mg/kg, and hair lead, 312 versus 80 mg/kg. For females, the mean results were slightly lower: 2.3 versus 1.7, and 149 versus 50, respectively. Nemenko and Goncharov (344) have reported elevated levels of cadmium and lead in hair and blood as functions of air pollution levels and distance from the source. They also reported a sixfold decrease in the mercapto group of the exposed population. This may indicate binding of the heavy metals to sulfhydryl group on the blood proteins.

Hartwell *et al.* (345) have made a comprehensive study of the relationships between smelters and the deposition of lead, cadmium, and arsenic in both environmental and biological media. This multiple-media study included air, soil, household dust, tap water, food, blood, hair, and urine. The greatest exposures and the highest body burdens were found closest to the smelters, and, of the tissues and fluids sampled, hair was found to be the most useful in determining relationships between environmental metal levels, distance, and body burden. Wibowo *et al.* (346) have also conducted a multiple-media study and concluded ''measurements of lead in blood and of the zinc protoporphyrin in blood levels appear to be better biological parameters to assess both environmental exposure and health risk than measurement of lead in hair alone'' (p. 275).

Jervis and Tiefenbach (347) reported that children living in the vicinity of a gold refinery had a mean hair concentration of 6.7 ppm arsenic compared to 0.33 for the controls. Drinking water contaminated with arsenic from the smelter was suggested as the source of exposure. Mitoma *et al.* (348) reported arsenic levels as high as 3.4 ppm in the hair of those living near a refinery. Housworth (Morse *et al.*, 225) found urinary arsenic levels were positively correlated with water consumption and distance from the copper smelter in children who lived in the area. Hair arsenic levels, on the other hand, did not show these correlations. Ghelberg and Bodor (349), however, reported increased arsenic in the hair and urine of children and adults living around a copper refinery, and they (350) found hair analysis useful in screening for exposure to arsenic and other heavy metals. Bencko *et al.* (351) reported that the hair of children residing near a ferromanganese factory had twice the hair manganese concentration of control children (5.1 and 2.6 ppm, respectively).

The exposure of nonworkers to heavy metals from industries other than mining and refining has also been reported. Residents of an apartment complex were exposed to airborne arsenic when 75 kg of As_2O_3/Na_3AsO_3 dust was accidently released from a Dutch chemical factory (352). In this case, the analysis was able to differentiate between bulk and surface arsenic in or on the hair, and the contamination of the apartment residents was found to be the result of fallout, with little or no real intake of arsenic. In the Deutsche Demokratische Republik (East Germany), the hair and urine of children residing in a region with high airborne arsenic contained, respectively, 10 and 3 times more arsenic than did those of children from a control region (353). The corresponding hair and urine arsenic concentrations were 5.5 versus 0.5 ppm, and 0.011 versus 0.004 ppm, respectively. Bencko et al. (224) reported elevated blood, hair, and urinary arsenic in children residing in the vicinity of a Czechoslovakian coal-fired electricity generator. Obrusnik et al. (106, 354) have also established a relationship between the arsenic content of hair from the nonoccupationally exposed population and the emissions of coal-fired power stations, and they encouraged the use of hair analysis for an indicator of such environmental exposure. Johannesson et al. (355) have studied arsenic as well as cadmium, mercury, selenium, and zinc concentrations of hair in relation to volcanic and geothermal activity and found that these sources of pollution did not contribute to the body burden of heavy metals in the Icelandic population.

Industrialization and urbanization apparently increase the body burden of heavy metals. Significant differences in the metal concentrations of human hair have been reported for urban and rural populations. For example, Folio et al. (356) found that the hair of urban children had, on the average, one-quarter the arsenic, twice the lead, and four times the cadmium contents of children residing in the three adjacent rural Tennessee counties. The children in this study, unfortunately, were not age matched. All of the urban subjects were under 4 years of age, and all of the rural subjects were more than 4 years old. Mean ages were 2.4 and 11.3 years, respectively. In the Philippines, hair cadmium, mercury, and lead concentrations were not different for the urban and rural populations (357, 358). In South Korea, the cadmium concentration in hair from urban subjects was found to be twice that of the rural population (359).

Kim (360), however, has reported that the cadmium content of hair from army recruits living in Seoul did not reflect exposure to cadmium. Watanabe et al. (361) found that the cadmium and lead concentrations in the hair of Japanese schoolchildren was not related to the concentrations of these metals in the urban atmospheres of three Hyogo Ken neighborhoods. Imahori et al. (362) were also unsuccessful in demonstrating a relationship between hair and atmospheric concentrations of trace elements in a Tokyo neighborhood. They suggested that blood, urine, and tissues "may reflect the trace element body burden more directly" (p. 180).

In Sri Lanka, differences in hair lead levels between the urban and rural populations were related to industrial growth and urban development, as well as to climatic conditions and automobile traffic patterns (363). Lux and Rauh (364) found the highest lead concentrations in the hair of those living along streets having the highest volume of automobile traffic in the German city of Hamm. Caccuri et al. (365) were unable to demonstrate significant differences in the hair lead levels of those living in different parts of Naples.

In Leipzig, however, hair lead levels were related to lead pollution of the urban atmosphere (366). The hair of dairy cows from some selected areas in the Erfurt district of the DDR did not show elevated levels of lead, even though the lead contents of their organs and milk were found to be slightly increased (367). In Czechoslovakia, the hair of deer from polluted and nonpolluted areas showed significantly different concentrations of lead as well as of arsenic and cadmium (368).

The hair of humans living in industrial and agricultural areas of Belorussia showed significantly different concentrations of lead, but not of arsenic, mercury, or antimony (369, 370). In Poland, significant differences in hair mercury levels were reported for residents of urban and rural areas (371) and of industrial and agricultural (372) regions. Similar significant differences for the hair lead levels have been reported for residents of different regions of Poland (373–375). The lead contents of hair from Yugoslav school-age children were reported to reflect lead pollution from automobile traffic (24), and Ahmed (376) will soon report the results of a study on lead pollution involving over 1000 schoolchildren from five regions of Saudi Arabia.

In addition to the airborne heavy metals, those in drinking water and food are serious sources of exposure outside of the occupational environment. While the likelihood of inhaling heavy metals from polluted air is high, the likelihood of ingesting them from contaminated food and water is even higher. The heavy-metal hazards are often discovered in ambient monitoring programs by public health agencies, but hair analysis has found frequent application in identifying such exposures. Elevated hair arsenic levels coupled with mild clinical symptoms of arsenic ingestion were traced to pollution by mine drainage in China (226), and elevated hair and urinary arsenic concentrations were correlated with high drinking-water levels of arsenic in Hungary (222). In the United States, hair and urinary arsenic concentrations showed clear relationships with the consumption of contaminated drinking water by residents of California (44) and Utah (377). Similar correlations between hair and urinary arsenic concentrations and the level of arsenic pollution of the drinking water have been made for exposed and unexposed populations in Mexico (220) and in Chile (221). From a subsequent study in Chile, Cortes *et al.* (378) concluded that the hair of the exposed population could serve as a sensitive monitor of water pollution by arsenic and mercury.

Valentine and her co-workers (379, 380) investigated the relationships between (a) environmental exposure to selenium in drinking water and (b) the selenium concentrations in blood, urine, and hair, and (c) glutathione peroxidase activity. Clemente and his research group (109; Cigna-Rossi *et al.*, 381) have carried out studies on the concentrations of selenium and mercury, as well as of other heavy metals, in the blood, urine, and hair from residents of several regions of Italy in relation to dietary and environmental factors. Uyeta *et al.* (382) have suggested reconsidering the significance of hair mercury concentrations because they did not observe a decrease in response to decreased mercury concentrations in unpolished rice following prohibition of mercurial pesticides in Japanese rice fields, but they did not consider other dietary sources of mercury.

The consumption of mercury-contaminated fish is perhaps the chief source of nonoccupational mercury exposure. Several relationships have been established between fish consumption and the concentration of mercury in the hair. In some cases, these are supported by correlations between measurements on the mercury concentrations of the fish and/or blood mercury concentrations of the consumer. Riolfatti (383) has investigated the mercury exposure of two Italian populations and found that the hair and blood mercury concentrations were correlated with the amount of fish consumed. The mean hair and blood mercury concentrations were 0.07 mg/L and 3.06 mg/kg, respectively. Gras and Mondain (384) have reported a similar study on Senegalese students and fishermen. The blood and hair mercury concentrations of the fishermen were found to be 0.035 and 7.33 ppm, respectively. In the Colony of Seychelles, where annual per capita fish consumption is 100 kg, Matthews (238) found correlations between the mercury contents of fish and the mercury levels of the hair. Lin (385) has reported that urinary and hair mercury concentrations were correlated with mercury intake for two groups of Chinese fishermen from islands off the coasts of the Shandong and Liauning Provinces. Silvalingam and Sani (386) found hair mercury concentrations of 8 ppm in the hair of Malaysian fishermen, but they were unable to establish a correlation between mercury in hair and mercury in fish. Suckcharoen et al. (387) have reported a localized increase in the mercury contents of fish and hair at the site of a recently established caustic soda factory in Thailand.

Kyle and Ghani have reported on two studies of fish consumption and mercury exposure. In the first (388), they established a firm correlation between hair mercury concentrations of Lake Murray residents and the consumption of fresh fish from Lake Murray. In the second (389), they were unable to correlate the hair mercury concentrations of the urban poor from Port Moresby with the mercury content of tinned marine fish. The Lake Murray population ate fish two or three times per day: Fish consumption was less in the Port Moresby group.

In Japan, several investigations (390–392) have established correlations between the fish-eating habits of the populations and the mercury contents of the hair. The last investigation (393) reported that males ate more fish and had correspondingly higher hair mercury levels. The hair mercury levels were reported to decrease in response to a change in the fish-eating habits of Japanese who emigrated to Brazil (393). The mean values, which also reflect the male–female differential, are listed in Table 6.4.

Dose–response relationships between frequency of eating fish and hair mercury level were found in four Japanese immigrant settlements in South America (393a). In a study of Brazilians, a mean hair mercury concentration of 3.36 ppm was determined, but no correlation between hair mercury concentration and shellfish consumption was established (394). In North America, Phelps et al. (395) found the concentration of mercury in hair was related to that of the blood for a population

Table 6.4 ▪ Mercury Contents of Hair of Japanese Immigrants to Brazil and Japanese Residents in Japan, ppm

	Brazil	Japan
Men	1.48	5.50
Women	1.39	3.49

known to have consumed large amounts of mercury-contaminated fish. The concentrations of mercury in the hair were 300 times greater than those in the blood. Harada et al. (396) reported a correlation between the mercury concentration of the hair and the quantity of fish in the diet for reservation Indians in Ontario. Neurological symptoms were observed in those with the higher (greater than 50 ppm) hair mercury concentrations.

In the United Kingdom (U.K.), duplicate diet studies (237, 397) have shown elevated hair and mercury levels in populations consuming mercury-contaminated fish. Hislop et al. (398) were able to measure mercury in the blood, scalp hair, and facial hair of 20 volunteers who had consumed known quantities of mercury-contaminated halibut for a 3-month period. The scalp hair mercury concentration rose to a maximum mean value of 25 ppm 130 days after the study began and then decayed to 5 ppm 3 months later. Scalp hair to blood mercury ratios ranged from 200:1 to 340:1 during the course of this study.

Contrary to findings for the British population, Den Tunkelaar et al. (399) found very low mercury concentrations in the hair of the Dutch population, and they concluded that hair concentrations were not an acceptable parameter to screen for mercury in the population. In the Finnish population, however, the consumption of mercury-contaminated fish is reflected in elevated hair mercury levels (400, 401). Hansen et al. (41) reported a firm correlation for mercury levels in the blood and hair and the consumption of seal. The mean blood level was 63 μg of mercury per liter. The correlation coefficient for hair blood and hair mercury concentrations was 0.9222, and the blood:hair mercury ratio was 1:289.

Airey (38) has demonstrated that hair mercury concentrations are related to fish-eating habits. She evaluated over 500 hair samples from 32 locations in 13 different countries and found hair mercury concentrations of 11.6, 2.5, 1.9, and 1.4 ppm for those who ate fish every day, every week, twice a month, and once a month, respectively. From a review of the literature, she (39) subsequently established a positive linear correlation between hair mercury concentration and fish consumption for some 7500 individuals in 35 countries:

Hair mercury concentration = 1.67 + 0.13 Fish consumption

where the hair mercury concentration is expressed in mg/kg and the fish consumption is expressed in kg/person/year.

The 1975 data of Creason et al. (91) show exposures of children to mercury and lead in the domestic environment. They found that the concentrations of these elements in scalp hair paralleled those of the household dust. Ten years later, Matsubara and Machida (402) concluded, "Hair can be regarded as a sensitive indicator of mercury contamination" (p. 236). Recently, Limic and Valkovic (403) have reported the development of mathematical models for using hair analysis to evaluate environmental heavy-metal exposures. Hair analysis can certainly be used to evaluate heavy-metal exposures in the occupational and domestic environments. And it is valuable in screening for such exposure, but clinical observations and testing are necessary for confirmation of heavy-metal absorption.

7

Collection and Preparation of Hair Samples

The initial step in hair analysis is the collection of the hair sample. This is followed by the physical and/or chemical procedures required to prepare the sample for the determination of its trace element contents. Sample collection practices have ranged from the uncontrolled snipping of distal ends in barber shops and beauty salons to the random selection of predetermined numbers of hairs from specified regions of the scalp, with careful alignment of the proximal ends. Sample preparation almost always involves some kind of washing procedure to remove surface dust and dirt. Subsequent treatments depend upon the techniques employed for the trace element determinations, such as weighing and encapsulation prior to neutron activation analysis (NAA) or digestion with acids to destroy the organic matrix prior to atomic absorption spectrometry (AAS).

The popularity of hair analysis has been due, in part, to the ease with which samples may be collected. Until recently, however, there has been little agreement on the when and where of sample collection. The trace element composition of human hair has been shown to vary with both time and location. As a recording filament, hair is extruded from the body at a rate of approximately 0.3 mm/day. The trace element composition in the more distal regions are more likely to be affected by the external environment than are those of the more proximal regions of the hair shaft. Similarly, the trace element concentrations in hair from exposed surfaces of the body are more likely to be affected by these external factors than are those of the hair from surfaces of the body that are usually covered by clothing. It is important to consider these factors in interpreting the results of hair trace element determinations.

7.1. Anatomical–Longitudinal Variations of Trace Elements in Hair

Some information on the variations of hair trace element concentrations with respect to anatomical location was presented in Section 2.2. With a few exceptions, there appears to be a consensus that the trace elements in or on human hair have both endogenous and exogenous components and that the exogenous component varies with the anatomical location. Growth rates may also affect the apparent concentrations for some of the macroelements. Varier et al. (65), for example, reported that the calcium concentrations in axillary hair and facial hair were $3\frac{1}{2}$ and $1\frac{1}{2}$ times higher, respectively, than the concentrations of calcium in scalp hair. The more rapid growth of the scalp hair could be considered as a diluting factor to reduce the calcium concentration.

Varier et al. (65) have also reported variations in the concentrations of some of the macroelements in scalp hair from one individual on the basis of sampling sites. They found twice as much chlorine in hair taken from the "right front" as they found in hair taken from the "back top" of the scalp. Similarly, they found twice as much calcium in a hair sample from the "left front" as they found in a sample from the "back bottom" of the same scalp.

Seta et al. (404) have also investigated variations in the elemental composition of hair with respect to the location on the scalp from which the sample was collected. They divided the scalp into five regions: frontal, vertex, nape, left lateral, and right lateral. Five hairs were collected at each site from each of 12 Japanese males. A 0.5-cm segment taken at 3 cm from the proximal end of each hair was examined by scanning electron microscopy/energy dispersive x-ray analysis (SEM/EDAX) after each hair was washed and ashed. Site-to-site differences in calcium concentrations were as low as 25% from left lateral to right lateral for one of the subjects to as high as almost 300% from right lateral to vertex for another.

While the scalp hair concentrations of calcium, and possibly other elements, appear to show site-to-site variations, there is no evidence that the hair from any one site is always of higher or lower concentration than the hair from any other location on the scalp. The occipital region of the scalp is the most frequently cited location for the collection of hair samples. The nape of the neck is also popular as a site for the collection of hair samples.

The concentrations of trace elements in scalp hair have also been reported to show longitudinal variations. Some of these were described in Section 2.1. These variations usually show gradual increases in the concentrations of trace elements in progressing from the proximal to the distal end of the hair. This has been attributed to exogenous deposition, which increases as exposure of the hair to the external environment increases. A rise in the concentration of a toxic element, followed by a decline, is usually interpreted as indicative of an acute exposure. With the development of instrumentation for automatic scanning and measuring along the length of the hair and of software for applying mass density corrections to the results, longitudinal distributions of both toxic and essential elements are now determined as a matter of routine (52, 405–407). Bos et al. (66, 408) have developed a system for measuring trace element concentrations across the diameter of the hair; this system shows promise as a means of differentiating between elements of endogenous origin and those of exogenous origin. The longitudinal variations have led to some agreement on using the "proximal inch" for the determination of trace element concentrations in human scalp hair when the assessment is directed to the current or most recent period. Otherwise, long strands of hair are considered as recording filaments for the assessment of trace element depositions during the recent past.

7.2. Recommended Sampling Protocols

One IAEA (International Atomic Energy Agency) protocol on activation analysis of hair as an indicator of contamination of humans by environmental trace element pollutants calls for the collection of at least 100 individual hairs taken 5 to 10 strands at a time from 20 to 10 (respectively) different sites on the scalp (409).

Each hair strand should be clipped close to the scalp (within a few millimeters). The distal and proximal ends should be identified. It is recommended that as a rule 10 cm of the strand should be left for the routine analysis, cutting off the distal end. However, a length of 5 cm may be used for individuals with short hair. In order to make measurements of 10 cm long hair comparable with those of 5 cm long hair, the 10 cm strands should be cut in two halves to be analysed separately. Similar considerations are valid for strands of 15, 20, etc. cm length. The hair should be cut with clean plastic scissors. If a metallic tool has to be used, oxides must be carefully removed, and a few millimeters must be cut off from both ends of each strand. using a plastic or quartz tool under laboratory conditions. From the head of each individual not less than 100 strands should be collected, 5–10 from each of 20–10 [respectively] different 2–4 mm² spots, evenly distributed over the head. . . . The total weight of the 5 cm samples is typically 10–100 mg. But if the time, technique, labour and expense make it admissible, separate determinations for the different spots (around 5 mg each sample) would be desirable. . . .

Scalp hair of man is divided into five regions as follows:
  1. frontal
  2. temporal
  3. vertex anterior
  4. vertex posterior
  5. nape

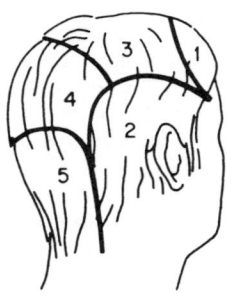

A more recent IAEA protocol from a coordinated research program on the significance of hair mineral analysis as a means for assessing internal body burdens of environmental mineral pollutants requires only a single cutting from the occipital region (410).

The Hair Analysis Standards Board (32) has also recommended a procedure for collecting samples.

This section promulgates recommendations for gathering human hair specimens for trace element analysis.

1 The Board strongly recommends that all hair specimens be collected under direct professional supervision, either in the office of a health professional or by a person trained in proper techniques for hair specimen collection. If a hair specimen has not been collected under professional supervision or by a properly trained person, that fact should be stated on the submittal form and the final laboratory report since contamination may invalidate the results.

2 Because the preponderance of published data listing norms and reference ranges for elemental concentrations in hair deal specifically with nape-of-the-neck hair, the Board recommends that whenever possible hair specimens should be collected from the nape of the neck. The portion of the scalp from which a hair specimen is collected should be stated on the submittal form and the final laboratory report. Hair from other portions of the scalp may be used, when so noted on the report, but only with the recognition that clinical interpretation may be somewhat less significant. The hair submitted should represent the first 1 to 2 inches of recent growth from the scalp and should not include long ends.

3 In the absence of scalp hair, other body hair such as beard hair, axillary hair, or pubic hair, may be analyzed. It must be fully recognized, however, that published data for such hair are inadequate for accurate interpretation. It has been suggested that hair from areas other than the scalp may be useful in distinguishing between exogenous contamination of scalp hair as opposed to internal absorption of toxic elements.

4 Sample size should range from 500 milligrams to 1 gram, depending upon the technology used, and the sample size should be obtained from at least 5 and preferably 10 or more separate locations along the nape of the neck. Hair specimens should be cut as close to the scalp as possible and should be limited to the first 5 centimeters of recent growth.

5 Whenever possible, instruments used to cut hair specimens should be made of plastic, quartz, or some other suitable material which will not contaminate the hair specimen. Further research is necessary to determine which types of cutting instruments will not contaminate the hair specimen. This information is especially needed by the hair analysis industry so that recommendations can be made to physicians using hair analysis services in their practices. Until alternate instruments are available, cutting instruments made of high-quality, surgical-grade, stainless steel may have to be used.

6 Contamination from the hands or gloves of personnel collecting hair specimens should be avoided as much as possible. In practical terms, in a clinical setting, this is best done by washing and drying the hands before collecting a hair specimen. Further research is necessary to determine whether gloves should be worn during the collection procedure, and if so, what type of gloves. Again, the hair analysis industry, in particular, needs this information so that it can make recommendations to practitioners about the best way to avoid contamination from the hands or gloves of personnel collecting hair specimens and thereby introducing significant error into the analytical results.

7 As a final comment on collection procedures, the Board reminds all personnel involved in hair analysis of the importance of meticulous general housekeeping, including the elimination of such sources of contamination as dust or other environmental contaminants; and the need for careful handling of hair specimens before packaging for shipment. A representative sample of each lot of containers to be used for shipping hair specimens should be tested before use to eliminate the possibility of introducing contamination from the shipping containers. As an example of potential contamination, some hair shipping envelopes with an adhesive flap have been licked with saliva and sealed with hair trapped beneath the adhesive material. This practice may introduce potential elemental contaminants from three sources: saliva, the adhesive, and exposure to the external environment.

The description of sampling sites found in the literature include terms such as "occipitonuchal" region, "suboccipital" region, "verticoposterior" region, and "neckenpartie." The sampling procedures have been described as "during hair cut," "randomly over scalp," or "cut close to the scalp." While by no means universally adopted or accepted, the many samples appear to have been collected by cutting the hair at the nape of the neck or back of the head, close to the scalp, with stainless steel scissors. Usually, several hundred milligrams is sufficient sample for most trace element determinations. Such samples are conveniently stored in plastic vials or envelopes made from plastic sheet.

7.3. Washing Procedures for Removing Exogenous Trace Elements

While it seems quite reasonable to remove dust, dirt, and other surface contaminations from the hair sample by washing it prior to the determination of its trace element contents, Chittleborough (35) and others (411) have suggested "that a no-wash, holistic approach to hair sampling and analysis can be realistically adopted to obtain valid information concerning associated endogenous and exogenous trace elements." Chittleborough argued that "a knowledge of the separate contributions of both endogenic and exogenic sources may prove to be quite valuable to the environmental scientist," while recognizing that "those concerned with human biology may be essentially interested in the levels of endogenous trace elements in the hair" (p. 71).

The classical works of Bate and Dyer (49) and of Kopito and Shwachman (23) recognized the need for and the possible consequences of washing the samples prior to trace element determinations. The former observed that washing either with an acetone–alcohol mixture, followed by rinsing with water or with a dilute aqueous solution of a nonionic detergent, followed by rinsing with water, removed most of the sodium but only small percentages of the copper, manganese, and zinc from the hair. The latter found that boiling water removed sodium, potassium, calcium, magnesium, and chlorine from the hair while allowing full recovery of lead. On the basis of radiotracer studies and electrochemical studies respectively, Rakovic and Pilecka (411a) and Pilecka *et al.* (411b) have concluded that calcium losses from hair to aqueous washing media are insignificant (<5%).

Subsequently, Assarian and Oberleas (412) compared the removals of copper, magnesium, and zinc from a pooled hair sample by three cleaning procedures: (a) soaking in an aqueous solution of sodium lauryl sulfate (SLS), (b) soaking sequentially in hexane, ethanol, and water, and (c) soaking sequentially in acetone, diethyl ether, acetone, and SLS solution. Their results are summarized in Table 7.1. They questioned the reliability of hair as a diagnostic tissue on the basis of the sensitivity of its trace element contents to the washing procedure.

Jervis *et al.* (104) found that sequential washing with water, ethanol, and diethyl ether reduced the zinc concentration to 89.0% of its unwashed value, but they consider losses of up to 20% negligible. Chattopadhyay *et al.* (8) have used this

Table 7.1 ▪ Removal of Some Trace Elements from Hair by Various Washing Procedures[a]

Washing procedure	Percentage retained		
	Cu	Mg	Zn
None	100	100	100
a. SLS solution	76.0	39.8	91.3
b. Hexane–ethanol	87.1	42.9	98.8
c. Acetone–ether	55.0	44.7	97.5

[a]After Assarian and Oberleas (412).

water–alcohol–ether washing procedure to prepare hair samples for lead analysis. On the basis of replicate pre- and postwashing analysis of 11 different samples, they found that from 83.7 to 100% of the lead was retained in the hair. Ryan *et al.* (413) reported that the pre- and postwashing concentrations of zinc were the same, and the postwashing copper concentration was 95% of its prewashing value, but 20% of the bromine, calcium, and manganese were lost during the water–ethanol–acetone washing procedure, as was 40% of the gold and chlorine.

For removing external contamination prior to the determination of hair cadmium concentrations, Ellis *et al.* (322) used a multistep cleaning process consisting of sequential agitations of the samples in acetone, acetone, water, water, detergent solution, detergent solution, water, and acetone. Each step in the process was monitored by scanning electron microscopy and electrothermal AAS; exogenous cadmium was assumed to be removed by this process. Salmela *et al.* (414) have evaluated four washing agents for removing contamination from three different hair samples. They concluded that both the washing agent and the duration of washing were important considerations, but they were unable to establish when washing was complete and when the leaching of endogenous trace elements began.

Kumpulainen *et al*, (415) have also evaluated four different washing agents, and they concluded that a hexane rinse followed by two 20-minute washes with aqueous SLS solution was suitable preparation prior to the determination of endogenous chromium. Mattera *et al.* (416) have reported that 78% of the exogenous copper was removed from the hair by 5% aqueous sodium dodecyl sulfate (SDS) at neutral pH, and they concluded that only such mild washing conditions were acceptable for hair sample preparation. Clanet *et al.* (53) reported that exogenous copper and zinc were not removed by sequential washing with acetone, water, and acetone. And Fergusson *et al.* (74) found that the tendency of the hair to absorb exogenous trace elements increased from manganese to zinc to copper. The sequential washing with acetone, water, and acetone, however, has been reported to remove endogenous cadmium (417). Washing with diethyl ether alone removed more mercury than sequential washing of the same samples with diethyl ether and an aqueous solution of a nonionic detergent (38). These results are partially reconstructed in Table 7.2. Niculescu *et al.* (235) have used scanning electron microscopy to confirm that

Table 7.2 ▪ Effect of Washing Procedures on the Mercury Contents of Human Scalp Hair[a]

Washing procedure	Mercury contents, ppb	
	Sample G	Sample R
None	88 ± 6	586 ± 23
Triton-X 100	80 ± 1	506 ± 40
Ether	76 ± 5	496 ± 11
Ether–Triton	82 ± 5	568 ± 41

[a]After Airey (38).

sequential double washings in acetone, ether, and aqueous solutions of SLS removed all surface particulates from the hair prior to the determination of its lead contents.

Chatt *et al.* (418) have made a comprehensive study of the effects of six washing procedures on the concentrations of a dozen and a half elements in an in-house reference hair. Some of their results are summarized in Table 7.3, and these show (a) that little if any mercury was removed by any of the procedures, (b) that the major portions of the lead and arsenic were removed by all of the washing procedures, and (c) that all of the washing procedures increased the manganese con-

Table 7.3 ▪ Comparison of Washing Procedures on the Trace Element Contents of Hair[a]

Element	Washing procedure, mean element concentration (SD), ppm				
	Unwashed	A/W/W/W/A[b]	Aq. SDS[c]	Aq. T-X 100[d]	E/W/A/[e]
Aluminum	23.8 (2.6)	9.34 (0.29)	6.21 (0.73)	7.80 (0.83)	6.99 (0.75)
Arsenic	0.276 (0.015)	0.031 (0.01)	0.044 (0.02)	0.020 (0.01)	0.072 (0.02)
Bromine	14.7 (0.77)	6.63 (0.58)	5.48 (0.34)	5.24 (0.33)	9.13 (0.32)
Calcium	2008 (54)	1715 (63)	1532 (49)	1575 (55)	1668 (36)
Chlorine	325 (15)	155 (7)	141 (30)	124 (23)	200 (18)
Cobalt	6.70 (1.64)	0.128 (0.02)	0.110 (0.01)	0.119 (0.04)	0.127 (0.003)
Copper	21.4 (1.35)	19.9 (1.06)	20.6 (2.60)	22.2 (1.90)	21.5 (2.75)
Lead	4.94 (0.39)	0.375 (0.04)	0.436 (0.04)	0.407 (0.04)	0.489 (0.05)
Manganese	0.98 (0.08)	1.29 (0.12)	1.76 (0.03)	2.70 (0.40)	1.80 (0.54)
Mercury	2.36 (0.19)	2.37 (0.19)	2.32 (0.22)	2.21 (0.20)	2.40 (0.22)
Selenium	1.21 (0.15)	1.03 (0.23)	1.08 (0.20)	0.98 (0.23)	1.01 (0.13)
Zinc	220 (5.6)	209 (7.3)	197 (5.3)	207 (3.3)	217 (9.2)

[a]After Chatt *et al.* (418).
[b]A/W/W/W/A = sequential washings in acetone, water, water, water, and acetone.
[c]Aq. SDS = washed with an aqueous solution of sodium dodecyl sulfate and rinsed with water.
[d]Aq. T-X 100 = washed with an aqueous solution of Triton X-100 and rinsed with water.
[e]E/W/A/ = sequential washings in ether, water, and acetone.

tents of the hair sample. These results may be interpreted as demonstrations of (a) the endogenous nature of the mercury, (b) the significant exogenous contributions to the lead and arsenic contents of the hair, and (c) the contamination of the sample with manganese during the washing procedure, respectively.

Ohmori (314) found that sequential washings in acetone, water, and acetone removed lesser amounts of the trace elements from hair than did washing with 1% aqueous caledathamil solution. The data presented by Suzuki *et al.* (419) show that sequential washings in acetone, water, and acetone removed lesser amounts of the trace elements from hair than did washing with 1% aqueous SLS solutions or with a 1% aqueous solution of a polyethoxyether. Buckley and Dreosti (420) have studied the removal of exogenous zinc from human hair and of endogenous zinc from rat hair by aqueous solutions of edathamil, SLS, and polyethoxyether with the aid of radiotracer zinc. Very little exogenous zinc was removed from human hair by water or by 1% aqueous Triton X-100. Almost all of the exogenous zinc was removed from the human hair by 1% SLS, 1% disodium ethylenediamine, and 0.05% nitric acid solutions. The aqueous SLS, disodium ethylenediamine, and the nitric acid solutions removed endogenous zinc from the rat hair more actively than did water or aqueous Triton X-100 solution. On a subject-by-subject basis, Thiery *et al.* (421) found no differences in the copper concentrations of unwashed hair and hair sequentially washed in acetone, water, and acetone. De Groot *et al.* (293) found, on the other hand, that the sequential washing of hair with acetone, water, and acetone reduced its aluminum concentration by approximately fourfold, relative to unwashed hair. Das *et al.* (422) reported that sequential washing of hair with acetone, water, and acetone removed only small amounts of copper, zinc, and mercury, and that significant amounts of cobalt, chromium, and iron were removed by this treatment. Ryabukhin (409) has tabulated some two dozen preirradiation treatments used to clean hair prior to the determination of trace elements by NAA. Pankhurst and Pate (423) have included information on which of a dozen different washing procedures was used to prepare the hair samples they cite in their exhaustive tabulations of hair trace element concentrations.

7.4. Recommended Cleaning Procedures

The aforementioned sequential washing with acetone, water, and acetone is the procedure currently recommended by the IAEA (410). While it is probably adequate for the removal of surface dust and dirt, there is no confirmation that it will efficiently remove exogenous trace elements from the hair while leaving the endogenous trace elements completely undisturbed. The IAEA Coordinated Research Programme (CRP) protocol is as follows:

> Wash hair (tied in a lock) successively in acetone, thrice in water, and once more in acetone. (Acetone should be of reagent grade and water of highest purity.) Add sufficient amounts of the

above solvents to cover the sample entirely. At each wash, allow the sample to stand at room temperature for 10 min in contact with the solvent with constant stirring. After each wash, decant the liquid and add fresh solvent. (A procedure that can be used as an alternative to and/or in combination with the described washing method is the utilization of the ultrasonic bath.) Carry out the washing in a dust free enclosure (e.g., glove-box, laminar flow hood.)

The Hair Analysis Standardization Board (32) clearly recognized the many problems associated with cleaning hair samples prior to the determination of their trace element contents. For this reason, their recommendations on laboratory hair-washing procedures presently lacks firm guidance. It is expected that the following procedures will undergo significant modification.

This section contains tentative recommendations for washing hair samples before the digestion procedure and testing. The recommendations are for commercial laboratories that do such tests. The Board urgently requests that research results and practical experience from various laboratories be provided to the Board for use in refining these recommendations. The Board recognizes that much more scientific research must be done before more definitive recommendations can be made.

1 Normal hair hygiene procedures, such as frequency of shampooing, should be followed up to the time the specimen is collected. Product names of hair treatment preparations, frequency of use, and last date of use should be recorded on the submittal form and in the final laboratory report. A hair sample should not be taken until 10 weeks after a cold (permanent) wave or bleaching treatment, and then only the first $2\frac{1}{2}$ centimeters of recent hair growth (that closest to the scalp) should be gathered for analysis.

2 Hair analysis laboratories should provide clients with a complete list of hair preparations known to contain high concentrations of elements which could affect the final analytical results. The submittal form and final laboratory report should show frequency of use and time lapse from last use of all such preparations.

3 Weighing hair samples before washing them eliminates the possibility of contaminating the washed sample during the weighing procedure. This technique requires, however, that weighing, washing, drying, and digestion be performed in the same container to prevent the possible loss of hair during the wash procedure. Most laboratories, therefore, weigh the sample after washing the hair. This requires scrupulous handling to avoid contaminating the washed sample during the weighing steps. Whether the specimen was washed before or after it was weighed should be stated in laboratory reports.

4 The Board recognizes that the scientific literature on hair washing techniques is extensive and often conflicting. The extremes are represented by 1) an organic solvent wash followed by a detergent wash and water rinse and 2) a detergent wash and water rinse. The Board agrees unanimously that further research on this subject is definitely needed. The general (but not unanimous) consensus of the Board was that tentative recommendations for hair specimen washing procedures should include:

    a. An organic solvent such as (but not limited to) acetone or ethanol, followed by:
    b. an aqueous wash.

5 All aqueous solutions used for trace element analysis should be prepared from deionized or distilled water meeting NCCLS Type I Standards (National Committee for Clinical Laboratory Standards Approved Standard: ACS-3, "Specifications for Reagent Water Used in the Clinical Laboratory"; NCCLS, 771 E. Lancaster Avenue, Villanova, PA 19085). Water and all solutions used for preparing the hair sample for analysis should be tested and found free of trace element contamination at the time of preparation and use.

7.5. Procedures for Dissolving Hair Samples

Dissolution of the hair sample may be necessary in order to complete the measurement of its trace element contents. A wide variety of dry and wet ashing procedures are available when this is the case. Friel and Ngyuen (410a) have evaluated some of these techniques, and they recommend dry ashing of hair samples to be analyzed for copper, manganese, and zinc and wet ashing with nitric acid for iron assays. Difficulties are rarely encountered in applying any of the standard procedures for dissolving biological tissues to hair samples. The absence of lipid materials in the washed hair samples usually makes them easier to dissolve than most other biological tissues. Some of these procedures for dissolving the hair sample, along with their corresponding sampling sites, washing procedures, and techniques for measuring trace element contents, are listed in Table 7.4.

The Hair Analysis Standardization Board (32) has made recommendations on the digestion of, and the subsequent trace element determinations in, hair samples, but these provide little guidance for the actual digestion procedures:

This section contains standards for hair digestion and the analytical determination of element concentration in the digestant.

1 Any techniques or equipment used, even as a technique in which a very small specimen, such as individual hairs or portions of individual hairs can be analyzed, must measure elemental concentrations of a homogenous digestate of a 500 milligram sample or larger, obtained from at least five different locations on the scalp, preferably the nape. Because elemental concentrations vary so widely from hair to hair and from segment to segment of individual hairs, a sample of at least 500 milligrams from a minimum of five separate locations is required for significant clinical interpretations.

2 No laboratory shall report any measurement when the measurement falls below the detection limit, or level, for that laboratory with the method used. The detection limit is defined by the American Chemical Society (ACS) in "Guidelines for Data Acquisition and Data Quality Evaluation in Environmental Chemistry," *Analytical Chemistry,* Vol. 52, No. 14, December, 1980, pages 2242–2249. Because hair analysis is a screening test, this Board recommends that the detection limit be defined in terms of two times the standard deviation of the "noise" obtainable by the method used, rather than three times the standard deviation of the noise, which the ACS requires for more precise analysis. The mere fact that a value is below or above the detection limit, as defined above, does not necessarily mean that the person from whom the hair specimen was obtained is deficient or has an excess of that element. Many other variables must be considered.

3 Each hair analysis laboratory should list its own detection limits in hair, as defined above, for every element reported and on every report.

4 The Board further recommends that every hair analysis laboratory report its results in the same standardized units of parts per million (ppm) or, micrograms per gram ($\mu g/g$), of dry weight contained in the original sample.

Table 7.4 ▪ Survey of Sample Sites, Washing Procedures, Dissolution Procedures, and Measurement Techniques for the Determination of Trace Elements in Hair

Sample site	Washing procedure	Dissolving procedure	Measurement technique	Reference
Back of head	7-X-OMATIC	Nitric/perchloric	Atomic absorption	T-131
Nape of neck		Nitric acid	Atomic absorption	T-132
Above each ear	None	Perchloric/peroxide		T-133
Occipital region	Nonionic detergent	None	Neutron activation	T-134
Occipital region			Atomic absorption	T-135
Occipital region	Nonionic detergent	Perchloric/peroxide	Atomic absorption	T-136
Occipital area	SLS solution, then acetone, then ether	Dry ash, 1 N HCl	Atomic absorption	T-137
Nape of neck	"SNOOP"	Dry ash, HCl	Emission spectro.	T-138
Nape of neck	SLS solution, ether	Dry ash, HCl	Atomic absorption	T-139
Occipital area	Heptane, alcohol, water	Dry ash, nitric	Atomic absorption	T-140
Occipital region	Nonionic detergent, petroleum ether	Nitric/perchloric	Atomic absorption	T-141
		None	Neutron activation	T-142
Occipitonuchal region	Acetone, ether, SLS solution	Nitric/perchloric	Atomic absorption	T-143
Occipital portion	Nonionic detergent	None	Neutron activation	T-144
Back of head	Nonionic detergent	None	Neutron activation	T-145
Back of head	Nonionic detergent	None	Neutron activation	T-146
Back of head	Nonionic detergent, alcohol, water	Nitric/perchloric	Atomic absorption	T-147
Verticoposterior	Unwashed	Char	PIXE	T-148
Random distal ends	Ether, water	None	Neutron activation	T-149
Neckenpartie	Acetone, water	None	Neutron activation	T-150
Neckenpartie	Acetone, water	None	Neutron activation	T-151
During hair cut	Nonionic detergent	Dry ash	X-ray fluorescence	T-152
Crown or nape	2% acetic acid	None	X-ray fluorescence	T-153
Nape of neck	0.1 M EDTA	Nitric/perchloric	Atomic absorption	T-154
Suboccipital area	Acetone, water	Nitric acid	Atomic absorption	T-155
Nape	Water	None	Neutron activation	T-156
Suboccipital area	Acetone, water	None	Neutron activation	T-157
Nape	Nonionic detergent	Nitric/perchloric/peroxide	Atomic absorption	T-158
Back of head		Sulfuric/peroxide	Atomic absorption	T-159
Randomly over scalp			Cold vapor atomic Absorption	T-160
Nape of neck	Water, carbon tet.	Nitric/perchloric	Atomic absorption	T-161
Occipital area	Detergent, alcohol	Nitric acid	Atomic absorption	T-162
Occipital region	Acetone, water	None	Neutron activation	T-163
Randomly over scalp	Water, acetone	None	Neutron activation	T-164

(*continued*)

Table 7.4 ▪ (*Continued*)

T-131.	Vivoli, G., Bergomi, M., Fantuzzi, G., del Dot, M., Tonelli, E., Zanetti, F., and Gatto, M., 5. Spurenelementensymposium Proceedings, Jena, July, 1986, pp. 509–514.
T-132.	Kohrs, M. B., Choh, K. H., and Nordstrom, J. W., Nutrit. Res., 1986, 6, 889–903.
T-133.	Gallagher, M. L., Webb, P. R., Crounse, R., Bray, J., Webb, A., and Settle, E., Nutrit. Res., 1984, 4, 577–582.
T-134.	Gibson, R. S. and DeWolfe, M. S., Nutr. Rep. Internat., 1980, 21, 341–349.
T-135.	Weijie, C. and Songguang, R., Kexue Tongbao, 1984, 29, 693–695.
T-136.	Hunt, I. F., Murphy, N. J., Cleaver, A. E., Faraji, B., Swendseid, M. E., Coulson, A. H., Clark, V. A., Laine, N., Davis, C. A., and Smith, J. C., Amer. J. Clin. Nutr., 1983, 37, 572–582.
T-137.	Dorea, J. G., Almeida, I. S., Queiroz, E. F. O., and Horner, M. R., Ecology of Food and Nutrition, 1982, 12, 1–6.
T-138.	Strain, W. H., Steadman, L. T., Lankau, C. A., Berliner, W. P., and Poris, W. J., J. Lab. Clin. Med., 1966, 68, 244–249.
T-139.	Reilly, C., Proc. Nutr. Soc. Australia, 1981, 6, 141–143.
T-140.	Gershoff, S., McGandy, R., Nondasuta, A., Pisolyabutra, U., and Tantiwongse, P., Amer. J. Clin. Nutr., 1977, 30, 868–872.
T-141.	McKenzie, J. M., Amer. J. Clin. Nutr., 1979, 32, 570–579.
T-142.	Bowen, H. J. M., Sci. Total Environ., 1972, 1, 75–79.
T-143.	Klevay, L. M., Amer. J. Clin. Nutr., 1970, 23, 284–289.
T-144.	Gibson, R. S., Sci. Total Environ., 1984, 39, 93–101.
T-145.	Gibson, R. S. and DeWolfe, M. S., Amer. J. Clin. Nutr., 1979, 32, 1728–1733.
T-146.	Gibson, R. S. and DeWolfe, M. S., Pediat. Res., 1979, 13, 959–962.
T-147.	Valentine, J. L., Kang, H. K., and Spivey, G., Environ. Res., 1979, 20, 24–32.
T-148.	Clayton, E. and Wooller, K. K., IEEE Trans. Nuc. Sci., 1983, NS-30, 1326-1328.
T-149.	Katz, S. A., Bowen, H. J. M., Comaish, J. S., and Samitz, M. H., Brit. J. Dermatol., 1975, 92, 187–190.
T-150.	Mende, T., Wiesener, W., Franke, W., Domschke, S., and Gorner, W., Isotopenpraxis, 1984, 20, 301–303.
T-151.	Wiesener, W., Gorner, W., Niese, S., Baldauf, K., Grund, W., Hennig, M., and Mende, T., Isotopenpraxis, 1981, 17, 278–282.
T-152.	Bacso, J., Kovàcs, P., and Horvàth, S., Radiochem. Radioanal. Letters, 1978, 33, 273–280.
T-153.	Basco, J., Lusztig, G., Pal, A., and Uzonyi, I., Exp. Pathol., 1986, 29, 119–125.
T-154.	Medeiros, D. M., Pellum, L. K., and Brown, B. J., Nutr. Res., 1983, 3, 51–60.
T-155.	Mazzotta, D. and Guarneri, M., Il Farmaco, 1986, 41, 397–403.
T-156.	Ward, N. I. and Minski, M. J., (University of London Reactor Centre) personal communication, 1984.
T-157.	Marumo, F., Tsukamoto, Y., Iwanami, S., Kishimoto, T., and Yamagami, S., Nephron., 1984, 38, 267–272.
T-158.	Capel, I. D., Pinnock, M. H., Dorrell, H. M., Williams, D. C., and Grant, E. C., Clin. Chem., 1981, 27, 879–881.
T-159.	Barlow, P. J., Sylvester, P. E., and Dickerson, J. W. T., J. Ment. Defic. Res., 1981, 25, 161–168.
T-160.	Pritchard, J. G., McMullin, J. F., and Sikondari, A. H., Brit. Dent. J., 1982, 153, 333–336.
T-161.	Raghupathy, L. and Sharma, V. N., Sci. Total Environ., 1985, 41, 73–78.
T-162.	Weber, C., Nelson, G., de Vequere, M., and Pearson, P., Nutr. Rep. Intern., 1984, 30, 1009–1018.
T-163.	Houtman, J., de Bruin, M., de Goeij, J., and Tjioe, P., *Nuclear Activation Techniques in the Life Sciences 1978*, Internatonal Atomic Energy Agency, Vienna, 1979. pp. 559–614.
T-164.	Obrusnìk, I. and Bencko, V., Radiochem. Radioanal. Letters, 1979, 38, 189–196.

8

Determination of Trace Element Levels in Hair

In considering the analytical techniques for the determination of trace element levels in hair, sensitivity and selectivity are of major significance, and factors such as speed, simplicity, cost, dynamic range, and multielement capabilities are important. While no single technique fully satisfies all of these criteria for every element, atomic and nuclear spectrometry and electroanalytical chemistry have been frequently applied to such determinations. Atomic absorption spectrometry (AAS), inductively coupled plasma atomic emission spectrometry (ICP/AES), x-ray fluorescence (XRF) spectrometry, charged particle-induced x-ray emission (PIXE) spectrometry, spark source mass spectrometry (SSMS), neutron activation analysis (NAA), and anodic stripping voltammetry (ASV) are among those that have been successfully applied to the determination of trace element levels in hair.

8.1. Neutron Activation Analysis (NAA)

For many years, NAA has enjoyed a favored position among the techniques used to determine the trace element composition of hair. This technique usually requires minimum sample preparation, and it usually allows several trace elements to be determined simultaneously. For NAA, sample handling can usually be reduced to collection, washing, drying, weighing, and encapsulation. Each laboratory has developed its own optimum sequence of conditions for radioactivation and postactivation measurement of the trace elements in hair. In practice, NAA is usually carried through at least two neutron irradiation–decay–measurement cycles for multielement determinations. The gamma spectra of the short-lived nuclides are recorded for a few minutes after irradiation and decay periods of a few minutes each. The spectra of the long-lived nuclides are recorded for perhaps an hour after several days or weeks of decay, following neutron irradiation periods of from hours to days.

One typical investigation on the concentrations of two dozen trace elements in human scalp hair from South Africa (481) began with washing the samples for 30 min in a 50/50 (v/v) acetone/water mixture, followed by drying for 2 days at 50–60° C. Duplicate specimens weighing between 10 and 80 mg were encapsulated in polyethylene and quartz containers for short- and long-term neutron irradiation. Standards were similarly prepared and coirradiated with the hair specimens. For the determination of aluminum, chlorine, potassium, manganese, sodium, and vanadium, the specimens and standards were irradiated individually under reproducible conditions for exactly 15 min, and the gamma spectra were individually recorded under reproducible conditions exactly 3.5 min after irradiation. For the determination of gold, bromine, cerium, cobalt, chromium, iron, mercury, potassium, lanthanum, sodium, antimony. scandium, and zinc, a 3-day neutron irradiation, followed by a 30-day decay preceded the measurement of the gamma spectra.

A somewhat different sequence of irradiation–decay–measurement cycles was used in Canada to determine some two dozen trace elements in scalp hair samples (413). The samples were washed twice for 5 min in water, using ultrasonic agitation. The samples were dried for 3 hours at 60° C (after which presumably they were weighed), sealed in polyethylene envelopes, and placed in irradiation vials. Three sets of standard irradiation, decay, and measurement conditions were selected. For selenium and silver, these were 30, 10, and 60 sec. Irradiation, decay, and measurement times of 10 min, 1 min, and 10 min, respectively, were selected for the determination of iodine, bromine, manganese, magnesium, copper, vanadium, chlorine, aluminum, calcium, and sulfur. And for the determination of barium, strontium, gold, zinc, arsenic, antimony, sodium, and potassium, these times were 3 hours, 1 hour, and 1000 sec, respectively. The neutron irradiations and the spectrum measurements for the samples and for the appropriate standards were performed under reproducible conditions.

It is possible to increase the sensitivity and selectivity of NAA by chemically isolating the element or elements of interest from the irradiated sample prior to recording its gamma spectrum. Czauderna (424) has developed a procedure for the radiochemical separation of selenium, silver, gold, antimony, platinum, mercury, cobalt, nickel, iron, zinc, molybdenum, tin, chromium, cadmium, copper, and arsenic from sodium, potassium, cesium, and rubidium by extraction with a zinc amalgam. Czauderna compared this procedure to the determination of some of these elements by the totally instrumental technique.

Wiesener *et al.* (263) have used a combination of radiochemical and instrumental NAA for the determination of two dozen trace elements in human scalp hair. The samples were collected from the nape of the neck, washed once in acetone, three times in water, and once again in acetone, dried for 2 hours at 80° C, and weighed into polyethylene tubes and quartz ampules. Fluorine, selenium, silver, aluminum, iodine, and manganese were determined by gamma spectrometry after brief (30–120 sec) irradiation and decay periods. Manganese, copper, and zinc were determined by gamma spectrometry after 1 hour of neutron irradiation and following removal of the sample from the quartz ampule with nitric acid. After 1, 20, or 50 hours of neutron irradiation, bromine, gold, chromium, antimony, zinc, iron, iridium, selenium, silver, and cobalt were determined by gamma spectrometry following the chemical separation of sodium with hydrated antimony pentoxide.

Biso et al. (425) have developed a radiochemical NAA procedure for the determination of mercury in human hair. Hair samples weighing 0.2 g were irradiated in quartz ampules for 8 hours at a thermal flux of $2 \times 10^{13}/cm^2$ sec. After an 8-hour decay, the contents of the ampules were opened, treated with appropriate carriers, and dissolved in a mixture of nitric and sulfuric acids. The chemical yield was determined by titration with ammonium thiocyanate, and the precipitated mercury thiocyanate was recovered for measurement of the hair mercury content by gamma spectrometry. The sensitivity of the procedure was 0.001 µg for a 200 mg hair sample, or 0.005 ppm. This is some threefold lower than the 0.01 –0.02 ppm detection limit claimed by Pritchard and Saied (426) for the determination of mercury in beard shavings by instrumental NAA.

Das et al. (427) have developed rapid and sensitive procedures for the determination of arsenic, antimony, and selenium in hair, based on neutron activation and radiochemical separation by mineralization with a saturated magnesium nitrate solution, followed by evolution of the hydrides and their absorption on active carbon. The determinations were then made from the gamma spectra of the carbon absorber, with detection limits of 10 ng. Bayat et al. (428) have also determined the arsenic concentration of hair by radiochemical NAA. They washed the hair samples successively in ether, acetone, water, and ether, and then 150 mg specimens were sealed in polyethylene containers. The hair specimens and standards were irradiated for 3 hours at a thermal neutron flux of $3 \times 10^{13}/cm^2$ sec. After decaying for 20 hours, the irradiated specimens and standards were treated with arsenic carrier and dissolved with nitric and sulfuric acids and hydrogen peroxide. The resulting solutions were introduced to cation exchange columns, and the arsenic contents of the effluents were determined by gamma spectrometry. The detection limit was 0.01 ppm.

The zinc, copper, and manganese contents of 10 hair samples were determined by both NAA and AAS (97). The hair samples were collected from the nape of the neck and sequentially washed with acetone, water, water, water, and acetone. Specimens of the hair samples and standards were encapsulated and irradiated for 1 hour at a thermal flux of approximately $5 \times 10^{13}/cm^2$ sec. Their gamma spectra were measured after removal from the irradiation capsule, and the zinc, copper, and manganese contents of the hair specimens were determined relative to the standards. For the AAS, 0.1 g specimens of the washed hair samples were dry ashed at 550° C, and the residues were dissolved in 0.1 N hydrochloric acid. The zinc, copper, and manganese contents of the hair specimens were determined from the atomic absorbances when aspirated into the air–acetylene flame. The results of this comparison are summarized in Table 8.1.

8.2. Atomic Absorption Spectrometry (AAS)

Selectivity and sensitivity, coupled with simplicity and low cost, make AAS the most widely used technique for the determination of trace elements in hair. But

Table 8.1 ■ Trace Elements in Human Scalp Hair, Comparison of NAA and AAS[a]

Sample number	Zinc		Copper		Manganese	
	NAA	AAS	NAA	AAS	NAA	AAS
1	221	201	11.4	11.1	5.3	5.0
2	119	100	34.7	36.6	13.1	11.3
3	147	150	23.0	22.9	0.5	0.5
4	244	230	10.2	10.6	8.9	11.5
5	173	154	9.2	9.0	1.1	1.4
6	131	128	8.9	9.6	1.6	2.1
7	136	139	10.2	12.5	0.3	0.3
8	212	210	23.9	25.3	1.1	1.6
9	202	204	23.3	18.1	0.4	0.5
10	218	203	30.4	34.2	4.3	5.2

[a]After Wiesener and Schaefer (97).

AAS suffers from the tedium of laborious sample preparation, and this technique lacks simultaneous multielement capabilities. Nonetheless, AAS has served as the basis of many investigations on the determination of trace elements in hair.

Harrison et al. (429) employed AAS to determine copper, iron, magnesium, and zinc in human scalp hair. Samples were collected from the nape of the neck and cut into 1-cm lengths to ensure homogeneity. The hair was then washed for 30 min in 1% nonionic detergent solution and rinsed with water. After drying overnight at 110° C, 0.5 g specimens were weighed into 50-ml Erlenmeyer flasks and treated with 5 ml of nitric acid. The acid was allowed to react slowly at room temperature to prevent foaming. The contents of the flask were then heated and treated with 1 ml of perchloric acid. The digestion was continued until dense, white perchloric acid fumes were evolved. At this point, digestion was complete. The contents of the Erlenmeyer flasks were transferred to 5-ml volumetric flasks and diluted with water. The copper and iron concentrations of the resulting solutions were determined directly, and those of zinc and magnesium were determined after further dilution by aspiration into the air–acetylene flame and measurement of the absorbance relative to standard solutions.

Nechay and Sunderman (430) have used this procedure for collecting, washing, and digesting hair samples prior to determining their nickel contents by AAS. The digested hair sample, however, was treated with ammonium pyrrolidine dithiocarbamate (APDC) to form chelates with the nickel and other transition metal ions, which were then extracted into methyl isobutyl ketone (MIBK). Aspiration of the organic extract into the air–acetylene flame improved the detection limits for the determination of nickel.

Salgado et al. (431) have also used the APDC–MIBK chelate extraction procedure to improve detection limits in the determination of trace elements in hair by AAS. Their samples were exposed to carbon tetrachloride vapors for 10 minutes, immersed in aqueous detergent solution (Tween 80) with occasional agitation for 10 min, washed with distilled water, immersed in 50/50 (v/v) ethyl alcohol/acetone solution for 10 min, and dried at 50° C. Half-gram samples were weighed into digestion tubes, treated with 3 ml of nitric acid, and heated for 30 min at a temperature of 150° C. After this time, 0.5 ml of perchloric acid was added, and the heating was continued for 1 hour at a temperature of 250° C. The contents of the digestion tubes were diluted to 10 ml. Five-milliliter aliquots from each tube were adjusted to pH 4.5 with aqueous ammonia, treated with 1 ml of 1% APDC solution, and extracted with 3 ml of MIBK saturated with water. After separation of the phases by centrifugation, copper, zinc, and lead were determined from the absorbances produced by direct aspiration of the organic layer into the air–acetylene flame.

Electrothermal atomization techniques have greatly increased the sensitivity of AAS. Bagliano et al. (432) employed this technique to determine cadmium, chromium, and lead in human hair. The samples were collected from the occipital region of the scalp, and the proximal centimeter was taken for analysis. Triplicate subsamples of 100 mg each were placed in teflon beakers and washed successively with magnetic stirring for 10 min in 125-ml portions of acetone, water, water, water, and acetone. The washed samples were allowed to air dry and equilibrate with ambient humidity overnight.

Two from each of the three subsamples were weighed into digestion vessels: Each third subsample was used to determine the moisture content of the hair so that results could be reported on a dry-weight basis. The contents of the digestion vessels were then treated with 3 ml of acid mixture made from 5 parts concentrated nitric acid + 1 part of concentrated perchloric acid. The digestion vessels were closed and placed in an oven maintained at 110° C for 45 min. The contents of the digestion vessels were transferred to 100 ml polypropylene volumetric flasks and diluted with high-purity water. Triplicate, 20 µl injections were made from each flask into the graphite tube atomizer, and optimized drying, charring, and atomizing times and temperatures were used to determine each of the trace elements. Sensitivities for cadmium, chromium, and lead corresponded, respectively, to 0.08, 0.9, and 3.0 µg of metal per gram of hair. Using similar pressurized digestion vessels and samples of human hair from the Commission of the European Communities (CEC), Voellkopf and Grobenski (433) determined arsenic, cadmium, lead, and selenium at concentrations of 0.2, 0.5, 30, and 2 ppm, respectively, with the stabilized temperature platform furnace and Zeeman background correction.

Baseline concentrations of manganese in hair were also measured by flameless atomic absorption spectrometry with Zeeman background correction (434). Samples were collected from healthy, dark-haired males aged 30 to 45 years. The hair was cut as close to the scalp as possible from random areas of the head, and the samples were washed and dried by the aforementioned procedures of Harrison et al. (429). Half-gram specimens of washed and dried hair were weighed into pressure decomposition vessels and treated with 5 ml of nitric acid and 2 ml of sulfuric acid. The vessels were closed and heated for 40 min at 140° C. After cooling for 30 min, the digestion vessels were opened, and their contents were transferred to polypropylene graduated flasks and diluted to 50 ml with high-purity water. An autosampler was used to make replicate 20 µl injections of the digested hair specimens containing standard additions of manganese into the graphite tube. The mean and standard deviation for replicate measurements on samples from 15 individuals were 0.26 ± 0.05 µg of manganese per gram dry hair.

Cold vapor atomic absorption spectrometry has been successfully applied to the determination of mercury in hair. Nord *et al.* (435) successively washed hair samples with ether, acetone, and SLS solution and then rinsed them with water, acetone, and ether. Air dried, 30-mg subsamples of hair were weighed into 250-ml, wide-mouth Erlenmeyer flasks and treated with 10 ml of sulfuric acid, 1 g of potassium permanganate, and 15 ml of nitric acid. The samples were allowed to digest at room temperature for 2 hours. After this time, the contents of the flasks were diluted to 125 ml with water. The excess permanganate was destroyed with hydroxylamine, and mercury vapor was produced by treating the contents of the flasks with stannous chloride solution. The mercury vapor was then swept with air through a drying tube to the absorption cell of the atomic absorption spectrometer where the atomic absorption was measured. Peter and Strunc (436) have eliminated the nitric acid from the digestion procedure and developed a semiautomated analysis for mercury in hair by on-stream generation of the cold vapor. Suzuki and Yamamoto (437) have used cold vapor AAS to demonstrate the long-term stability of methyl mercury in human hair. The results of mercury determinations in human hair by cold vapor AAS show excellent agreement with parallel measurements made by XRF spectrometry (438) and with those obtained by radiochemical NAA (439, 440).

8.3. Proton-Induced X-Ray Emission (PIXE) Spectrometry

Flame AAS has been compared to PIXE spectrometry for the determination of trace elements in human scalp hair (441). Hair samples were collected from 40 workers known to be occupationally exposed to toxic elements. The concentrations of calcium, manganese, nickel, copper, and zinc in these samples were measured by both PIXE and AAS. The ratios of the mean results obtained by PIXE spectrometry to those obtained by flame AAS, with the standard deviations, were as follows:

Element	PIXE:AAS	Standard deviations
Calcium	0.92	0.11
Manganese	0.96	0.16
Nickel	0.94	0.31
Copper	0.96	0.25
Zinc	1.19	0.15

The conclusion from this comparison was that PIXE spectrometry was a feasible technique for the rapid, large-scale screening of hair samples.

When compared to NAA, however, PIXE spectrometry was shown to be somewhat limited in terms of the number of elements determined (442). The PIXE measurements were made on the dried residue from 1 drop of the solution resulting from the digestion of 26 mg of hair in 1 ml of nitric acid. With the exception of the results obtained for calcium, agreement between the two techniques was good, and PIXE was better suited to the determination of lead. Baptista et al. (443) have compared the results obtained by PIXE from hair targets prepared in two different ways: eight matched hair strands mounted in an aluminum frame versus the residue from a drop of the solution resulting from the digestion of the hair in nitric acid. Their samples were collected and washed by the IAEA procedures cited in Section 7.2, and their results for copper, iron, and zinc are summarized in Table 8.2. They attribute the differences to "local elemental hair concentrations" in the solid samples and "average values" in the digested samples. Clearly, careful attention must be paid to target preparation procedures when PIXE spectrometry is employed for the measurement of trace elements in hair.

Pillay and Peisach (444) concluded that the PIXE spectrometry of hair could routinely be applied to environmental pollution studies from their measurements of calcium, iron, cobalt, copper, lead, bromine, iodine, and chromium in approximately 150 samples. The samples were first washed in ether and in acetone and then carried through two cycles of successive washings in water, 50/50 (v/v) acetone/methanol mixture, acetone, and ether. The cleaning was completed with a final ether rinse. Then each sample was frozen in liquid nitrogen and pulverized (known as "the brittle-fracture technique"). The pulverized hair samples were transferred to polymethyl methacrylate irradiation cells having Hostaphan windows

Table 8.2 ▪ Determination of Trace Elements in Hair by PIXE Spectrometry: Effect of Target Preparation Procedures[a]

Subject ID	Solid sample			Digested sample		
	Cu[b]	Fe[b]	Zn[b]	Cu[b]	Fe[b]	Zn[b]
Z-V-2-F	24	88	240	15	54	240
Z-V-7-A	18	13	140	99	180	580
Z-V-7-J	70	39	190	55	54	160
Z-V-6-A	23	27	360	18	95	170
Z-V-2-H	17	20	240	22	54	230
F-I	26	48	170	35	29	230
Z-V-5-H	37	95	350	44	11	400
F-E	60	56	510	51	75	470

[a]After Baptista et al. (443).
[b]Elemental concentrations of trace elements in hair in micrograms per gram.

for the measurements of their PIXE spectra. Their use of pulverized hair appears to have eliminated both some of the target geometry problems identified by Whitehead (445) and the need for acid digestion of the hair sample.

Mahrok et al. (446) have also used the "brittle-fracture technique" to prepare pulverized hair samples for PIXE spectrometry in their investigation of relationships between trace elements and mental retardation. Their samples were washed with 50/50 (v/v) acetone/ethanol prior to pulverizing them, and the pulverized hair samples were compressed into thin pellets for the measurement of their PIXE spectra. Hall et al. (447) and Paschoa et al. (448) prefer, however, to measure PIXE spectra from the residues of solutions obtained by acid digestion of the hair samples.

In addition to rapid, simultaneous multielement determinations in bulk hair samples, PIXE spectrometry has been successfully applied to the determinations of trace element profiles along the length of the hair shaft by automated longitudinal scanning techniques. Some of these were described in Section 7.1. Other applications of this technique are Henley et al. (449), Vis et al. (450), and Hong-Kou et al. (406).

8.4. Other Methods

Bacso et al. (279) have used both PIXE and XRF spectrometry (a) to evaluate the efficiency of washing procedures for hair samples, (b) to measure the calcium contents of the hair samples, and (c) to determine the longitudinal distribution of calcium in the hair samples. The PIXE measurements were found to be superior for the latter. Christensen (451) has used XRF spectrometry to determine simultaneously up to 20 elements, potassium through strontium, plus lead, mercury, gold, and cadmium, in hair samples, with detection limits ranging from 20 to 2 ppm. Wang (452) has also found XRF spectrometry reliable for the analysis of human hair.

Yurachek et al. (68) have applied SSMS to the determination of trace elements in human scalp hair. The hair samples were collected from the nape of the neck and washed with a 1% solution of a nonionic detergent in water prior to either dry or wet ashing. The residues from dry ashing were compressed onto support electrodes, or aliquots of the solutions obtained by wet ashing were evaporated in the presence of the electrode matrix and compressed onto support electrodes. The mass spectra were obtained from 100-μsec 30-kV sparks. The spectra were recorded on photographic plates, and the concentrations of 27 elements were determined from photodensitometric evaluations of the plates. Parallel measurements of magnesium, calcium, iron, copper, and zinc concentrations in one of the samples were made by AAS. The comparative measurements are summarized in Table 8.3.

Monasterios et al. (453) have demonstrated the analysis of hair samples for trace metals by ICP/AES without prior digestion. For this demonstration, the hair samples were collected during the course of normal hair cutting. They were washed by the IAEA procedure, and individual 10-mm-long hair segments contained in graph-

Table 8.3 ▪ Comparison of SSMS and AAS
for the Determination of Trace Metals in Hair[a]

	Mg	Ca	Fe	Cu	Zn
SSMS	16.4	135	2.72	16.2	246
AAS	21.8	210	8.72	17.7	236

[a]After Yurachek et al., (68). Values given in µg/g dry weight.

ite tubes were introduced to the plasma with a direct sample insertion device (DSID). Results for copper and zinc are compared to those obtained by direct aspiration flame AAS of samples prepared by acid digestion in Table 8.4. Chaudhri (454), Zhao (455), and Marquardt (456) have also made use of ICP/AES for the determination of trace elements in human hair.

Absorption spectrometry of metal ion complexes has also been applied to the determination of trace elements in hair. After destruction of the organic matrix by dry or wet ashing, the metal ion to be determined was selectively chelated, and its concentration was determined by absorbance measurements at specific wavelengths in the visible or ultraviolet regions of the spectrum. Singh et al. (457) have used pyrimidine-2-thiol for the determination of copper in hair after extraction of the chelate from alkaline media into MIBK and absorbance measurements at 400 nm. Wasey et al. (458) also used this reagent for the determination of copper in hair after extraction from aqueous media with molten naphthalene and dissolution of the solid in chloroform. Chen et al. (459) determined cobalt in hair from the absorbance of its chelate with 4-[(5-chloro-2-pyridyl)azo]-1.3-diaminobenzene in 12 M sulfuric acid, and Bing (460) used the absorbance of the tetra(4-trimethyl ammonium phenyl) porphyrin complex for the determination of mercury in hair. Chen et al. (94) determined selenium in hair from the fluorescence of the complex with 2,3-diammoninaphthalene in n-hexane.

Chittleborough and Steel (80) have measured the concentrations of zinc, cadmium, lead, and copper in hair by differential pulse ASV. Unwashed, 50-mg samples of hair were first predigested with 5 ml of warm nitric acid for 10 min, then treated with 5 ml of equimolar sodium and potassium nitrates, and evaporated to

Table 8.4 ▪ Comparison of ICP/AES with Flame AAS
for the Determination of Copper and Zinc in Hair[a]

Sample	Copper (ppm)		Zinc (ppm)	
	AAS	ICP/AES	AAS	ICP/AES
1	51.1	62.1	368	379
2	16.1	23.2	166	201
3	13.3	14.4	186	259

[a]After Monasterios et al. (453).

dryness under an infrared lamp overnight. The ashing was completed by furnace ignition at 400° C for 3 hours. The melts were dissolved in 5 ml of 0.15 M nitric acid and transferred to the electrochemical cell. The voltammetric procedure was carried out after adjustment of the pH to 4.7 with acetate buffer and displacement of oxygen with nitrogen. Typical results for a composite of facial hair were zinc, 173 ppm; cadmium, 1.84 ppm; lead, 4.20 ppm; and copper, 11.0 ppm. Dhaneshwar *et al.* (461) also used ASV for the determination of trace elements in hair. In 0.1 M potassium nitrate–0.1 M potassium chloride supporting electrolyte, they found hair concentrations of 140 zinc, 0.9 cadmium, and 58 ppm lead. Feher *et al.* (462) found lead and cadmium concentrations in hair from male and female subjects by ASV to be as follows:

	Lead (ppm)	Cadmium (ppm)
Male	54.7	5.5
Female	30.2	4.9

A variety of voltammetric techniques have been used for the determination of trace elements in hair. Polarography was employed by Meng and Zhao to measure zinc (463) and manganese (464). Zang (465) has determined selenium in hair by cathodic stripping voltammetry (CSV).

8.5. Selection of Analytical Techniques

There is no best or worst analytical technique for the determination of trace elements in hair. As mentioned, sensitivity and selectivity are of major significance. Whatever technique is employed must be evaluated with the appropriate reference materials, and a rigorous program of quality assurance and quality control must be applied to the entire analytical procedure.

9

Quality Assurance of Hair Analysis

Quality *assurance* differs from quality *control* in that the former involves an assessment of the overall process to ensure the *reliability* of the data while the latter is directed toward the routine activities associated with the *validity* of the laboratory results. Quality control procedures are usually included within the quality assurance program. A quality assurance program might include the following:

1. Project objectives
2. Organization
   a. Personnel
   b. Responsibilities
3. Sampling
   a. Collection
   b. Identification
   c. Preservation
4. Analysis
   a. Preparation
   b. Measurement
5. Instrument calibration standards
6. Quality control
   a. Reagent blanks
   b. Standards
7. Data reduction and reporting.

The project objectives and its organization are subject to considerable variability with respect to thrust and scope. It is, however, important that the personnel be trained and proficient in their specific tasks and that the quality assurance officer be actively involved in the planning, execution, and reporting of the project. Zlotkin (465a) has said, "For the practitioner, confidence in the accuracy of hair analysis reports and their interpretation for appropriate clinical application is still markedly lacking." Without a rigorous program of quality assurance and quality control, hair analysis is vulnerable to such criticisms.

9.1. Sampling

It has yet to be demonstrated that any specific area of the scalp is superior to any other with respect to sample collection. The general consensus appears to favor sample collection from the occipital or suboccipital region. The proximal inch or half inch is often used for subsequent determinations of trace element concentrations, but longer hair strands are required for the evaluation of their longitudinal distributions. Consistency in sample collection is necessary for quality assurance purposes. While this cannot be achieved on an interlaboratory basis, it can become established as the procedure within a laboratory or group of laboratories.

Consistency in sample collection includes not only the sampling site, but also the sampling instruments and the sample containers. These items should be carefully selected to preclude the introduction of contamination to the hair sample. Clean, dry scissors made from surgical-grade stainless steel and dry bags made from clean plastic sheet are suitable under most conditions. It is possible to estimate the potential for contamination during sample collection with blanks prepared by (a) using the stainless steel scissors to cut circles of filter paper into strips, and (b) storing the strips in plastic sample bags prior to trace element analysis. Comparisons to the results obtained from uncut, unstored filter paper circles would identify gross contamination introduced in the course of sample collection.

Documentation for sample identification must be initiated at the time of sample collection. The sample container must be labeled so that its contents can be unequivocally identified, and a permanent record must be made identifying the source of the sample and the conditions of its collection. The exact formats for labeling and recording may vary among laboratories, but this information is essential for correlating the levels of trace elements in hair with medical histories. dietary habits, or any other such parameters. The analytical results are useless without accurate sample identification.

Hair, unlike most other biological tissues, is stable. It does not require thermal or chemical preservation during storage. The sample container usually provides adequate protection from contamination, and the loss of endogenous trace elements from the hair shaft during storage is highly unlikely. Although hair samples can be stored in sealed containers under cool, dry conditions without preservation for extended periods of time, the analysis should not be delayed unnecessarily.

9.2. Analysis

It is necessary that the laboratory environment be scrupulously clean to avoid contamination of the hair sample, and that all laboratory manipulations be so designed that the potential contamination by or loss of trace elements is eliminated.

Contaminated glassware is a common source of error in trace element analysis. The following procedure is efficient for cleaning glass- and plasticware:

1. Scrub the glass- or plasticware thoroughly with detergent and water
2. Thoroughly rinse the glass- or plasticware with a solution of one part nitric acid to one part water
3. Rinse the glass- or plasticware with water
4. Rinse the glass- or plasticware with a solution of one part hydrochloric acid to one part water
5. Thoroughly rinse the glass- or plasticware with water
6. Thoroughly rinse the glass- or plasticware with deionized or distilled water of high purity
7. Allow the glass- or plasticware to dry in a dust-free environment. Dry the plastics at 50° C and the glass at 120°.

Contamination and loss are most likely to occur during the physical and chemical preparation procedures that precede the measurement of the trace element concentrations in hair. The traditional reagent blank is helpful in assessing contamination from acids or from fluxes used to dissolve the hair samples when this is necessary for the analysis. The blank, however, is of little value in assessing contamination due to the absorption of ionic or molecular species from the various agents used to wash the hair sample prior to digestion or ashing. The blank is also of no value in assessing the loss of trace elements from the hair sample during washing or dissolution.

The results of replicate analyses are useful in identifying contamination or loss, but such results rarely allow quantitative assessment of these errors. The addition of chemical spikes to specimens of the hair samples after the washing step sometimes allows the calculation of recoveries for the assessment of loss, but these corrections are always subject to question on the basis of chemical speciation. The inclusion of specimens of a standard reference material (SRM) or certified reference material (CRM) in the entire analytical procedure is the best approach to the evaluation of contamination and loss, as well as to the evaluation of precision and accuracy of the analysis.

The measurement of trace elements in hair is made in relation to appropriate reference standards, using their output signals to establish calibration of the measuring instrument. The instrument must be of adequate sensitivity and selectivity to generate suitable signals from the concentrations or masses of trace elements in the samples and standards. Operating conditions are established to optimize the output signals, and the output signals are monitored to ensure their stability and reproducibility. Frequent instrumental checks, as recommended by the manufacturer, are required for optimum operating efficiency. These may involve confirmation of parameters such as spectral location and detector response.

Heinonen (466) has reviewed the reliability of radiochemical and chemical trace analysis in environmental materials. Some of his methods for quality assurance are applicable to the determination of trace elements in hair. He urges the use of reference materials for assessing both the precision and the accuracy of the measurements, and he suggests replicate measurements on graded increments of these reference materials to identify "additive errors." The accuracy of the measurements can also be determined from analytical results obtained in various laboratories using various techniques. The assessment of accuracy is made from the relative total error (RTE):

$$\text{RTE} = e\% + 2(S\%),$$

where

$$e\% = 100(R - f)/R,$$

in which R is the reference value for the parameter measured, f is the amount found, and $S\% = 100$ standard deviation units.

The accuracy is excellent when the RTE is less than 25%, acceptable when the RTE is between 25% and 50%, and unacceptable when the RTE is greater than 50%.

The report of the IAEA's advisory group on quality assurance in biomedical NAA (467) also contains information relevant to the determination of trace elements in hair. The recommendations of the advisory group were summarized as the following checklist for quality assurance:

1. Obtain representative, uncontaminated samples;
2. Carefully avoid additions or losses of elements during sample storage and in the preparation of analytical samples ("clean" benches or "clean" laboratories may be necessary for analysis at ultratrace levels);
3. Optimize the analytical parameters (activation time, decay time, sample weight, position in the reactor, choice of detector, etc.) for the particular elements and matricies of interest;
4. Assess in advance whether RNAA must be employed, or preseparations, or whether INAA can provide equally good results;
5. Prepare accurate standards of the elements of interest rather than using certified reference materials as standards, and check that the decay-corrected specific activities are reproducible;
6. If radiochemical separation is employed, take pains that all sources of error associated with this step are minimized;
7. Monitor the analytical blanks and ensure that they are suitably low and reproducible;
8. Perform gamma ray spectrometry measurements and subsequent spectrum analysis carefully and promptly;
9. Analyze at least some of the samples in replicate, and compare the estimated overall precision with the observed variability, so as to ascertain whether any unknown sources of error are operating;
10. Check the accuracy of the overall analytical procedure by analysing certified reference materials of similar matrix compositions, and report the results obtained and the reference values used. (467, pp. 32–33)

9.3. Instrument Calibration

Instrument calibration is two-dimensional: It involves both selectivity and sensitivity. Spectrometry requires the accurate location of spectral position in terms of wavelength, energy, or mass for selectivity in identifying the trace elements. Calibration in this dimension is best achieved with individual standards for each element, prepared from high-purity materials. Mixed elemental standards should then be evaluated to determine if there are interferences in resolving the wavelengths or energies of the emitted or absorbed radiations from a specific elemental source. The sensitivity of the instrumental measurement is established from the signals generated by incrementally decreasing amounts of elemental standard in both the absence and presence of other elements. These calibrations must be reproducible to assure optimum selectivity and sensitivity. A part of the quality control is directed to the reproducibility of instrument calibration.

9.4. Quality Control

Among the commonplace quality controls are the reagent blank, the duplication of samples, the splitting and spiking of samples, the analysis of reference materials, the frequent reestablishment of instrument calibration, and the use of control charts. These controls are incorporated into the day-to-day laboratory routine for the determination of trace elements in hair.

For quality control purposes, reagent blanks in numbers equivalent to 5% of the hair samples undergoing analysis should be carried through the entire laboratory procedure. The concentrations of trace elements found in the hair samples should be at least 10 times greater than those found in the blanks, and the coefficient of variation for the blanks should be 10% or less. When these conditions are not met, the glassware cleaning procedure should be revised, and/or higher purity reagents should be used.

If the hair samples are sufficiently large, 10% of them should be carried through the entire laboratory procedure, from washing through measurement, in duplicate. The results from the duplicates should agree to within 10%. When this is not achieved, the quality assurance program must be reviewed to identify the fault.

After the preparation step, but before the measurement step, every tenth sample should be divided into two equal parts, and one of the parts should be spiked with known amounts of the trace elements expected to be present in the sample. The amounts of spike added should be equivalent to approximately half of the concentrations expected to be present. Recoveries of the spikes as determined from measurements on the spiked and unspiked specimens should be from 95 to 105%. Recoveries outside of this range may be due to matrix interferences.

Calibration of the measuring instrument must be confirmed frequently during the measurement procedure. This is conveniently achieved by including calibration standards as every tenth item in the measurement sequence. Modest adjustments may be made as needed, but significant changes in calibration usually signal the need to cease measurement and commence fault finding.

Control charts should be constructed from results obtained by replicate measurements on midrange calibration standards. The mean and standard deviation are calculated from a dozen or two results for such a standard, and either the two sigma limits or the 95% limits are used to establish upper and lower control limits around the mean. The midrange standard used to generate the data for the control chart is measured, along with the samples, in the course of future determinations, and the values obtained for this standard are plotted on the control chart. When a value for this standard exceeds either control limit, the analysis is out of control. No subsequent measurements are made until the fault is identified and corrected.

For its coordinated research program on the significance of hair mineral analysis as a means of assessing internal body burdens of environmental mineral pollutants, the IAEA (468) recommended the following procedures:

1. Inclusion of an analytical quality control material in every analytical run;
2. Analysis of "blind" analytical quality control materials provided by the Agency;
3. Results to be reported on RoA (Report of Analysis) forms;
4. Analysis of every sample in duplicate if the concentration value is less than 2× the limit of quantitation of the analytical method;
5. Analysis of occasional (e.g., every tenth) sample in duplicate if the concentration value is greater than 2× the limit of quantitation;
6. Occasional repetition of the whole validation procedure;
7. Retention of a duplicate sample for re-analysis should this be shown later to be necessary.

The IAEA further recommended the construction of control charts with 90% upper and lower control limits, using data from replicate analyses of reference materials and inclusion of these reference materials in the analytical scheme.

9.5. Reference Materials

In their recent survey of 100 reference materials, currently available from a dozen different national and international agencies and institutes, Muramatsu and Parr (469) have identified only 1 having a hair matrix. This material was prepared by Doctor K. Okamoto of the National Institute for Environmental Studies (NIES), Japan Environment Agency (470). Some 20 kg of human scalp hair was collected from three barber shops in Tsukuba and Tokyo. The hair was washed with 0.3% nonionic detergent in an ultrasonic cleaner, rinsed with copious quantities of distilled water, and dried overnight at 80° C. The dried hair was pulverized in an agate ball mill, sieved, blended, and packaged as individual 2-g units. The individual 2-g units were sterilized with 2 Mrad of ^{60}Co radiation. Certification of trace element concentrations in this material was based on results obtained by at least three independent analytical techniques. These certified values are listed in Table 9.1 as mean values with their two sigma limits. Some uncertified reference values are also listed in Table 9.1.

Suzuki et al. (471) have investigated this material by INAA. They determined the concentrations of 42 elements by gamma spectrometry after irradiation periods of 5 minutes and 5 hours. Their results are summarized in Table 9.2. The presence of high concentrations of silicon may be due to contamination from the agate ball mill used to pulverize the hair.

Table 9.1 ▪ Analytical Values NIES Reference Material No. 5, Human Hair[a]

Element	Mean ± 2	SD, μg/g
CERTIFIED VALUES		
Calcium	728	30
Iron	225	9
Magnesium	208	10
Zinc	169	10
Potassium	34	3
Sodium	26	1
Copper	16.3	1.2
Manganese	5.2	0.3
Mercury	4.4	0.4
Strontium	2.3	0.2
Nickel	1.8	0.1
Chromium	1.4	0.2
Cadmium	0.20	0.03

Element	Mean μg/g
REFERENCE VALUES	
Chlorine	250
Aluminum	240
Phosphorus	165
Bromine	90
Titanium	22
Lead	6.0
Barium	3.2
Selenium	1.4
Rubidium	0.19
Cobalt	0.10
Antimony	0.07
Scandium	0.05

[a]After Okamoto (470).

The human hair reference material, HH-1, was prepared by the IAEA for use in an intercomparison among laboratories participating in coordinated research programs on the elemental analysis of hair, sponsored by the agency (472, 473). This material was prepared from approximately 400 g of hair collected from several individual volunteers at the City General Hospital in Vienna. The hair was pulverized by the brittle-fracture technique, sieved through a 125 μm screen, blended, and tested for homogeneity. The resulting material was distributed, as 1-g samples, to more than 100 participating laboratories. The participants were requested to determine arsenic, cadmium, mercury, and lead as representative toxic elements, and chromium, copper, iron, and zinc as representative essential trace elements, in up to six replicate specimens of the sample, using those techniques with which the laboratories were most expert. The participating laboratories were also encouraged

Table 9.2 ▪ Analytical Results for NIES CRM No. 5, Human Hair

Element	μg/g	Element	μg/g
Sodium	26	Cadmium	0.23
Magnesium	220	Indium	0.007[a]
Aluminum	240	Tin	1.62
Silicon	12500	Antimony	0.073
Sulfur	49000	Tellurium	0.18[a]
Chlorine	250	Iodine	0.62
Potassium	36	Cesium	0.0141
Calcium	640	Barium	3.1
Scandium	0.046	Lanthanum	0.184
Titanium	22	Cerium	0.47
Vanadium	0.67	Niobium	0.30
Chromium	1.24	Samarium	0.0197
Manganese	4.7	Europium	0.0037
Iron	210	Terbium	0.0034
Cobalt	0.099	Dysprosium	0.023[a]
Nickel	1.73	Holium	0.34[a]
Copper	16.1	Ytterbium	0.025
Zinc	164	Lutecium	0.0019[a]
Arsenic	0.057[a]	Hafnium	0.0106
Selenium	1.29	Tantalum	0.0064
Bromine	92	Tungsten	0.041[a]
Rubidium	0.157	Gold	0.0127
Strontium	3.5	Mercury	3.6
Zirconium	2.3[a]	Thorium	0.022
Molybdenum	0.12[a]	Uranium	0.004
Silver	0.095		

[a]Indicates "less than."

to determine whichever elements they chose, in addition to those representative of the toxic and essential elements. Sixty-six laboratories from 28 different countries reported 2666 individual results, 40% of which were obtained by INAA, to the IAEA. The results were statistically evaluated by the IAEA, outliers were rejected, and certified values were derived for 20 minor and trace elements. For the representative toxic and essential elements, the mean values and relative errors were as follows:

As	0.053	16	Cr	0.27	29
Cd	0.26	23	Cu	10.2	9
Hg	1.70	5	Fe	23.7	13
Pb	2.73	21	Zn	174	5.

Table 9.3 ▪ Comparison of AAS and INAA
for the Determination of Some Trace Elements
in Reference Hair HH-1 (Mean ± SD)[a]

Element	Reference value (ppm)	Found AAS (ppm)	Found INAA (ppm)
As	0.053 ± 0.008	bdl[b]	bdl
Cd	0.26 ± 0.06	0.52 ± 0.18	bdl
Co	6.0 ± 0.4	14.6 ± 1.3	12.4 ± 3.2
Cr	0.27 ± 0.08	2.7 ± 0.4	0.33 ± 0.28
Cu	10.2 ± 0.9	22 ± 3	bdl
Fe	24 ± 3	79 ± 10	66 ± 17
Hg	1.7 ± 0.9	bdl	1.6 ± 0.5
Mn	0.85 ± 0.11	1.3 ± 1.2	1.1 ± 0.3
Ni[c]	2.3 ± 1.1	2.7 ± 0.9	bdl
Sb	0.031 ± 0.007	bdl	bdl
Se	0.35 ± 0.03	bdl	0.26 ± 0.34
Zn	174 ± 9	192 ± 21	181 ± 26

[a]After Coetzee, P. P. and Pieterse, H., S. Afr. Tydskr. Chem., 1986, 39, 85–88.
[b]bdl = Below detection limit
[c]Nickel reference value is not certified by IAEA

Coetzee and Pieterse (474) determined 10 trace elements in HH-1 by both INAA and electrothermal AAS. Their results are compared to the reference values in Table 9.3.

The United States National Bureau of Standards (NBS) initiated the preparation of a hair SRM, but this project appears to have been terminated. Some preliminary values for cadmium, lead, and zinc were determined by isotope dilution mass spectrometry, IDMS, and by AAS (475) (Cd = 1.178 ± 0.0056, Pb = 28.32 ± 0.99, and Zn = 189 ± 1).

Both the IAEA HH-1 and the NIES No. 5 human hair reference materials had mean sulfur contents of 49,000 ppm. The zinc concentrations of these samples as well as of the NBS material were similar, but the iron concentrations in these three materials span a decade of values: 23.7, 161, and 225 ppm for the IAEA, NBS, and NIES materials, respectively. The broad ranges for normal values of essential micronutrients such as iron and copper cause some to seriously question the significance of hair trace element determinations.

10
The Significance of Hair Analysis

Currently, there is little doubt that the elemental composition of human scalp hair is determined, partially, by the external domestic, recreational, and occupational environments in which the donor has been knowingly and unknowingly exposed to a wide variety of chemical compounds. At present, it is equally certain that systemic intoxication with cadmium, mercury, lead, arsenic, and possibly other elements is reflected by elevations of their concentrations in the hair and in other tissues. Firm correlations between trace element concentrations in hair and the abnormal physiologies of various diseases have, however, not yet been established, and it has not been clearly demonstrated that a dietary deficiency of a particular essential trace element results in a depression of its normal concentration in human scalp hair.

10.1. Current Status

Among three factors that prevent the use of hair analysis for the diagnosis of disease and for the assessment of nutritional status, first is the failure to establish normal ranges of concentration for the various trace and minor elements in human scalp hair. Several tabulations for the normal concentrations of trace and minor elements in human scalp hair have been prepared. An IAEA document on the use of hair as an indicator of human contamination by environmental trace element pollutants (476) contained 368 normal values for 39 different elements. The excellent review article by Pankhurst and Pate (423) included 657 citations of the average values for the concentrations of 42 different elements in human scalp hair. In Jenkins's report to the United States Environmental Protection Agency on toxic trace metals in mammalian hair and nails (477), 431 reference values for 15 different elements in human scalp hair were tabulated. Iyengar (478) selected 269 mean concentrations for 14 trace elements in hair as a pilot study to establish reference values for this tissue, as well as for blood, milk, urine, and liver. He suggested that "elements such as Cu and Zn are absolutely essential for life and are homeostatically regulated. Therefore, under ideal conditions, their levels may be expected to fluctuate within narrow limits for a given species, thereby justifying the usage of normal levels" (p. 3).

Matsubara (479) has provided information on the trace metal contents of hair from the rat, guinea pig, and human. His values are listed in Table 10.1. Some of the normal values for copper and zinc (cited in the aforementioned tabulations) are listed in Table 10.2. These values are based on at least 50 samples from healthy men and women. Each sample population was homogeneous with respect to domicile.

Rather than define normal values from his pilot study, Iyengar (478) identified "frequent values" for several trace elements in human scalp hair. For copper, these frequent values were most often in the range of 15–25 ppm. The corresponding frequent values for zinc and iron were 150–250 and 30–60 ppm, respectively. Luderitz et al. (480) have also identified reference ranges for the concentrations of some trace elements in the scalp hair of adult males residing in the DDR. Their reference values for copper and iron fall below Iyengar's frequent values, but their zinc reference value is within the frequent values of Iyengar. The reference values and their border ranges are presented in Table 10.3.

Marlowe et al (481) have quoted the "theoretical normal ranges" for some trace and minor elements in human scalp hair established by Doctor's Data, Inc., in evaluating their data on trace and minor elements in hair from a mentally retarded population and from a control population. And Kamakura (482) has compared the data he collected for 21 elements in scalp hair samples from 1899 normal Japanese subjects to the reference values established by MineraLab Inc. These normal ranges

Table 10.1 ▪ Trace Element Contents of Hair from the Rat, Guinea Pig, and Human[a,b]

Element	Rat hair		Guinea pig hair		Human hair	
	Geometric Mean	Geometric SD	Geometric Mean	Geometric SD	Geometric Mean	Geometric SD
Aluminum	1.31	1.17	0.65	1.5	15	1.9
Bromine	21.3	1.10	20.5	1.2	5.7	2.0
Calcium	173	1.14	170	1.2	410	2.0
Chlorine	512	1.15	1100	1.2	870	2.2
Copper	10.1	1.14	8.5	1.1	9.0	1.4
Iron	6.3	1.50	14	1.1	10	1.8
Mercury	0.31	1.55	0.49	1.3	3.4	1.6
Iodine	3.38	1.13	1.1	1.6	0.51	2.0
Potassium	691	1.43	390	1.2	17	2.2
Magnesium	57.5	1.18	100	1.3	38	1.8
Manganese	0.29	1.19	0.39	1.6	0.44	2.0
Sulfur[b]	3.4	1.05	3.1	1.1	4.5	1.1
Selenium	0.80	1.04	0.6	1.4	0.69	1.6
Zinc	204	1.05	210	1.05	150	1.2

[a]After Matsubara (479).
[b]All values are expressed in ppm except sulfur, which is expressed as %.

Table 10.2 ▪ Copper and Zinc Concentrations in Human Scalp Hair: Means/Standard Deviations from Various Reference Sources

Elements	References			
	476	423	477	478
Copper	12.2/4.1**[b]	18.5/x[a]	11/11*	6.8/1.6
	16.2/6.2***	12.2/x**	23/35	16.2/6.2***
	12.6/x	18/13	25.7/28.1	9.6/4.8
	11.7/x	18/18	17.9/11	12.2/4.1**
	11/11*	24/22	13.9/x	22/x
	13.1/9.9	16/10	34.7/6.7	26.2/15
Zinc	147/x	177/x		138/44*
	138/44*	183/x**		140/70
	180/70	138/44*		255/76.5
	208/137	167/53		150/25
	221/156	165/28		142/x
	255/110	205/90		185/x
	183/59**	148/x		142/77

[a]x indicates that the standard deviation was not given.
[b]*, **, or *** indicates that the same values have been cited in two or more of these references.

and reference values are presented in Table 10.4. For all 21 elements, the ranges of observed values from the Japanese population exceeded the MineraLab reference values.

Recent studies by Ward et al. (483) have reported mean concentrations for many trace and minor elements in the scalp hair of a small, heterogeneous sample of Bulgarian subjects that were in agreement with the aforementioned normal or frequent values. This also appears to be the case in a study of copper, iron, and zinc concentrations in hair from 222 Zambian subjects (57), and in a study of copper, manganese, and zinc in hair from 86 Canadian geriatric females (484).

Paschoa et al. (448) have reported on the concentrations of some trace elements in the scalp hair from 51 male and 50 female adult Mexicans. The hair samples were collected and washed by the IAEA procedures, and the trace element concentrations were determined by PIXE. The mean iron results were 266 ppm for males and 557 ppm for females. The mean copper results were 56 and 58 ppm for males and females, respectively. For zinc, the mean concentration in scalp hair from the males was 512 ppm; the corresponding value for the females was 557 ppm zinc. The ranges of the results spanned two decades for all three elements. Turkstra et al. (63) reported a mean hair iron concentration of 430, with a standard deviation of 750 for healthy South African adults. Their corresponding values for zinc were 194 ± 68. By any of the foregoing criteria, the Mexican and South African populations seem to have abnormally high hair iron levels. Abnormally high hair zinc levels appear to be demonstrated by the Mexican population but not by the South African subjects. A population of 260 students from Bombay also demonstrated normal zinc and high iron concentration in their hair (108).

Table 10.3 ▪ Recommended Divisional Age-Dependent Reference Ranges for the Concentrations of Elements in the Scalp Hair of Adult Humans[a]

Element/age group (years)	Reference value (µg/g)	Lower limit range (µg/g)	Upper limit range (µg/g)
Aluminum			
20–25	6–7	3–4	11–13
<20/>50	7–10	4–6	13–18
Lead	3–4	1.7–2.5	5–6
Cadmium	0.23–0.27	0.1–0.15	0.45–0.55
Calcium			
15–35	550–800	250–350	1200–1600
35–55	430–550	200–250	900–1200
<55	320–430	180–200	550–900
Chromium	0.15–0.18	0.07–0.1	0.25–0.35
Iron			
25–45	20–23	11–13	35–40
<25/>45	23–27 (30)	13–18 (20)	40–45
Copper	8.5–10	7–8	11–12
Magnesium			
15–35	30–38	18–22	50–66
<35	23–30	11–18	40–50
Manganese	0.6–0.7	0.3–0.4	1.1–1.2
Titanium			
20–45	0.4–0.5	0.2–0.23	0.7–0.85
<20/>45	0.45–0.6	0.23–0.27	0.85–1.2
Strontium			
15–35	0.9–1.2	0.4–0.6	2–2.7
<35	0.6–0.9	0.25–0.4	1.3–2
Zinc			
15–30	180–190	140–160	210–220
30–45	180–155	140–115	210–190
<45	155–160	115–130	190–195

[a]After Luderitz et al. (480). The hair samples were washed first with chloroform and then with water. Dry 200–500-mg specimens were dissolved in nitric and perchloric acids; the resulting solutions were diluted to 5 ml, and the concentrations of the trace elements were determined by ICP/AES.

A second factor hindering a broader utilization of hair analysis is a lack of information on the mechanisms by which endogenous trace elements are incorporated into the hair. Some important information on this aspect of hair analysis was demonstrated in the aforementioned study with the 86 Canadian geriatric females (402). The samples were collected, washed, and analyzed according to standardized procedures. A quality control material, HH-1 (for which the cited copper value is wrong), was incorporated into the analytical scheme. The results from two sets of hair samples collected 10 weeks apart showed that the concentrations of copper,

Table 10.4 ▪ Normal Ranges for Trace and Minor Elements in Hair

Element	Doctor's Data[a]	MineraLab[b]
Calcium	204–712	200–600
Magnesium	29–137	25–75
Phosphorus	108–203	100–170
Sodium	346–1080	150–350
Potassium	42–430	75–180
Iron	21–50	20–50
Copper	17–67	12–35
Molybdenum	0.59–2.55	0.10–1
Manganese	0.62–1.97	1.0–10
Zinc	104–288	160–240
Chromium	1.03–3.23	0.50–1.50
Selenium	0.08–0.64	3.0–6.0
Lithium	not established	0.10–0.80
Nickel	1.80[c]	1.0–2.0
Cobalt	not established	0.20–1.0
Vanadium	—	0.50–1.0
Lead	15.0[c]	20–30
Mercury	3.0[c]	2.5–5.0
Cadmium	1.6[c]	1.0–2.0
Aluminum	2.9–82.5	20–40
Arsenic	0.4[c]	2.0–3.0

[a]Doctor's Data, Inc., Post Office Box 111, West Chicago, IL 60185.
[b]MineraLab, Inc., 22455 Maple Court, Hayward, CA 94541.
[c]Normally tolerated limit established by Doctor's Data, Inc.

manganese, and zinc did not change on an individual or a group basis, and that no significant correlations related either the hair and serum zinc values or the hair and serum copper values. These observations were interpreted as reflecting some individual variability in the homeostatic regulation, and it was suggested that very different time scales are reflected by the concentrations of trace elements in hair and in serum. Serum concentrations provide an "acute index" over a short time period, whereas the concentrations in hair provide a "retrospective index" of trace element supplies. It was concluded, on this basis, that the hair zinc concentration was regulated by one of the smaller, non-albumin-bound fractions of the zinc in serum such as that bound to α-2-macroglobulin or to amino acids. It was speculated that only a small fraction of the serum zinc could be involved in regulating the hair zinc concentration. Changes in serum zinc concentration were not, therefore, reflected as changes in hair zinc concentration. However, small concentration changes of nonessential heavy metals in serum or blood were readily reflected by dramatic changes in the heavy metal concentrations of the hair. This simple model adequately explains the observations of Medeiros *et al.* (485), who found that dietary zinc supplementation increased the concentrations of zinc in serum and urine but not in hair. This model also justifies the conclusion reached by Matsubara and Machida (402), "Hair can be regarded as a sensitive indicator of mercury contamination, as inorganic mercury appears readily in the hair and stays there for a long time" (p. 236).

That only a small fraction of the serum zinc could be involved in regulating the hair zinc concentration is consistent with Laker's (67) arguments favoring hair analysis for determining trace element levels in humans. He maintains that 75 to 85% of the blood zinc is associated with carbonic anhydrase. Under such conditions, it is unlikely that this important cofactor would be discarded to the hair. His enthusiasm for hair analysis is based on its advantages over blood, as follows:

1. Hair provides a better assessment of normal trace element concentrations because short-term variations are averaged out. By taking a length of hair equivalent to a few weeks' growth and measuring the bulk concentration, an average concentration over that period may be found.
2. Hair offers a good way of discerning long-term variations in trace element concentrations. This may be done by measuring the variations along the length of long hair equivalent to several months, or by taking samples periodically.
3. Unlike blood, hair is an inert and chemically homogeneous substance. The structure of hair is permanent and once a trace element atom is incorporated into it, it is fixed there.
4. The concentrations of most trace elements are relatively high in hair as compared to the rest of the body, especially blood.
5. Hair provides a record of past as well as present trace element levels.
6. Specimens can be collected more quickly and easily than specimens of blood, urine, or any other tissue. Specimens do not deteriorate and may be kept indefinitely without the need for special storage conditions. (67, p. 261)

He recognized the difficulties associated with evaluating the effectiveness of the various washing procedures and in determining whether or not such procedures remove any of the endogenous trace elements. He recommended further research to clarify any uncertainty about the absorption into the hair of zinc, selenium, and possibly thallium from shampoos and the elution from the hair of endogenous trace elements in the course of bleaching, dying, or other cosmetic treatments.

The difficulties in differentiating between such exogenous depositions and the trace elements deposited endogenously is the basis for the third factor impeding more comprehensive applications of hair analysis. Limic and Valkovic (403) have considered the incorporation of elements into the hair structure from air particulates, water, shampoos, and other media. They developed mathematical models for the concentration of an element within a single hair strand in terms of four parameters: body stores, genetic effects, body fluids, and environmental contributions. Assuming both cross-sectional and longitudinal homogeneity of the hair strand, they applied experimentally determined radial diffusion coefficients for lead, selenium, and zinc to the radial distribution of these elements, as it was described by a set of empirical equations for only the environmental contributions. The calculated cross-sectional distributions were in fair agreement with the profiles measured by micro-

PIXE spectrometry. This agreement inferred that it may be possible to predict the origin of trace elements in hair from their cross-sectional distributions.

Houtman et al. (486) suggested three different stages for the deposition of trace elements in the hair: (a) from the body via the blood during formation; (b) from the body via sebum and sweat after formation; and (c) from the external environment via air and water after formation. It was noted that hair could take up elements from aqueous solutions by a mechanical swelling process, as well as by diffusion and chemical bonding at active sulfhydryl and amino groups of the protein. It was also noted that trace elements could be washed out of hair. Penetration and desorption rates were attributed to the specific properties of the elements present in the sweat, sebum, air particulates, water, aqueous solutions of shampoos, cold wave agents, dyes, and so on, and to the pH of the medium. On the basis of cross-sectional distributions at the root and at 1 and 2 cm above the root, measured by microbeam-PIXE spectrometry and of bulk concentrations in these samples measured by radiochemical NAA, it was possible to distinguish between

a. Elements mainly introduced from the blood during the first phase of hair formation (Cu, Zn) . . .
b. elements also introduced from the blood in a somewhat later stage (K, Ca, Fe), and . . .
c. elements introduced from sebum or sweat after completion of hair formation (Pb, As, Se) (486, p. 206).

If this is the case, it would appear that the copper and zinc concentrations in hair are homeostatically regulated to the greatest extent, while those of lead, arsenic, and selenium are the least regulated. The concentrations of potassium, calcium, and iron would fluctuate as a result of secondary effects. This possibility may explain the aforementioned abnormally high iron concentrations in the hair of the South African (63) and Indian (108) populations.

Bos et al. (66, 408) have applied the proton microbeam to radial and longitudinal PIXE spectrometry of hair. The resulting concentration profiles for sulfur, copper, zinc, iron, potassium, and calcium have led to some interesting speculations on the incorporation of trace and minor elements into the hair. The sulfur profiles agree with the morphology of the hair shaft and show that keratinization was complete long before leaving the follicle. The copper and zinc profiles showed maxima at the external root sheaths, which indicated a transcellular source of these elements, in addition to the matrix and connective tissue papilla. The absence of strong correlations between hair and serum concentrations of these elements was attributed to their partial incorporation into the former tissue from the internal root sheath. The iron distributions showed strikingly high concentrations in the root sheaths. Although the transversal route seemed blocked, there was some evidence of radial input. This peaking of iron on the periphery was offered as an explanation of the deviations in its concentration. Potassium was localized in the hair bulb and associated with the metabolic activity of the follicle. The calcium concentrations increased longitudinally due to exogenous contributions and appeared to penetrate the medulla. At the distal ends, exogenous calcium could not be distinguished from endogenous calcium. At the proximal ends, however, the exogenous calcium was easily removed by washing the hair in boiling water.

10.2. Future Perspectives

The suitability of hair analysis as a means of screening for heavy-metal exposure and heavy-metal poisoning is well documented. The utilization of hair analysis for these purposes will necessitate the continual refinement and standardization of methods for the collection and preparation of hair samples so that the data can be successfully compared on an interlaboratory basis. More information is needed to better define normal values for the elements in human scalp hair. Iyengar's tabulations (478) must be supplemented with additional data from laboratories using standardized methodologies in order to confirm or negate the need for geographically based normal values. Standard reference materials (SRMs), in addition to those available from the National Institute for Environmental Studies (Yatabe-machi, Tsukuba, Ibaraki 305 Japan) (470), should be developed for the laboratory quality control of hair analysis.

Significant progress has been made on differentiating between endogenous and exogenous trace elements in hair by radial and longitudinal scanning micro-PIXE spectrometry using the proton microprobe. Vis (487) has undertaken several collaborations directed toward measuring endogenous calcium in facial hair, tracing protein-bound mercury in the hair root, and identifying the metabolically active forms of copper and zinc distributed between the liver and hair tissues. The results of these collaborations will be valuable in identifying the mechanisms by which endogenous trace elements are incorporated into the hair.

Tykva (488) is also investigating the mechanisms by which endogenous trace elements are incorporated into the hair. He has extracted protein-bound lead and mercury from the hair of rats injected with radiotracers of these heavy metals. The protein–metal complexes were separated by electrophoresis and characterized to identify the transport mechanisms of the heavy metals. Such pharmacokinetic data will be useful in relating the hair concentrations of heavy metals to their concentrations in other tissues.

The relationships between the concentrations of trace elements in human scalp hair and in other tissues are being studied by Matsubara (489) with respect to the (a) elemental distributions in healthy humans and animals, (b) elemental concentrations in the hair of polluted humans and animals, and (c) multielement analysis of human hair as a means of detecting multielement metabolic shifts in the body. One source of the multielement metabolic shift was attributed to metabolic abnormality or disease. In this respect, low concentrations of zinc in the hair were associated with malignant tumors. One possible outcome of this investigation may be an evaluation of multielement hair analysis for the diagnosis of disease.

The optimism of a decade ago was reflected in titles such as "Hair: A Diagnostic

Tool to Complement Blood Serum and Urine" (490), "Hair and Health" (20), and "Hair: A Monitor of Chemical Exposure and Disease" (21). At that time, it was proposed that

> While many laboratories enthusiastically accept the use of scalp hair as a biopsy tissue, several serious questions remain. Before trace element analysis in scalp hair becomes an acceptable diagnostic indicator of mineral metabolism, additional work is required in four specific areas: (1) normal values showing a narrow range must be established, (2) sample collection and sample preparation procedures must be standardized, (3) trace elements incorporated into the hair from within the body (endogenous) must be differentiated from contamination by external (exogenous) sources, and (4) standard reference materials must become available to allow laboratories to establish quality assurance programs (21, p. 14).

While these questions have been fully or partially answered, the utilization of hair analysis data for the diagnosis of disease has made little progress. In 1987, it was demonstrated that osteoporotic women had lower scalp hair calcium concentrations and higher blood calcium concentrations than age-matched, gender-matched controls from the same environment (491). In another 1987 report (492), samples from post-myocardial-infarction patients showed (a) a decrease in the scalp hair concentrations of copper, magnesium, strontium, and barium, and (b) an increase in the ratio of the scalp hair calcium concentration to the scalp hair magnesium concentration. Interest in hair analysis for the diagnosis of disease is, according to Muramatsu (493), expected to grow, but he warns, "The scientific basis for these diagnoses is, however, still largely lacking. Health authorities are necessarily becoming involved as a result of the demand for treatment of possibly non-existent diseases" (p. 1). Clearly, more fundamental research is needed on the role of trace elements in human diseases and their relationship to the concentrations of trace elements in human scalp hair.

If, as suggested by Houtman (486), the incorporations of copper and zinc into the hair are homeostatically regulated, hair analysis data should be applicable to assessing the nutritional status of these elements. The failures to demonstrate elevations of hair zinc concentrations in response to zinc supplementations to the diets of well-nourished subjects has been interpreted as being equivalent to observing reduced hair zinc concentrations upon dietary deprivations of this element. This is not necessarily true: The latter experiments must be conducted to determine (a) whether indeed dietary deficiencies of essential trace elements are reflected by their decreased concentrations in the scalp hair, and (b) whether subsequent dietary supplementation restores them to normal values. Thereby, hair analysis may be shown to be useful in the assessment of nutritional status.

The application of hair analysis to the detection of therapeutic and abused drugs in the human body is being developed as an alternate to urinalysis. The immediate advantages of hair over urine for the determination of drug residues are related to the permanency of hair as a recording filament, and to the stability of hair as a biopsy material. The drugs are assumed to be absorbed into the hair roots from the blood stream and incorporated into the protein structure of the hair matrix. The procedures currently available for drug residues parallel those used for trace elements and suffer the some concerns regarding the differentiation of endogenous from exogenous materials. The measurement of drug residue is frequently made by radioimmunoassay, and the Psychemedics Corporation of Santa Monica, California, is prepared to carry out the **r**adio**i**mmunoassay of **h**air (*hair* spelled backward) for drug residues on a commercial basis. Baumgartner and Jones (494) and Puschel *et al.* (495) have successfully applied RIAH to the detection of opiates and other drug residues.

10.3. Conclusions

The determination of trace elements in human scalp hair has become an accepted adjunct to the more traditional analyses of blood and urine for identifying systemic heavy-metal intoxication. The complementary aspect of hair analysis is its ability to record acute exposures from the recent past. Hair analysis has its obvious advantages for monitoring environmental exposures to heavy metals. Continued interest and activity in the use of hair as a biopsy material will establish the place of this approach as a probe for the evaluation of trace elements in the body.

References

1. Flesch, P., in *Physiology and Biochemistry of the Skin*, S. Rothman, ed., University of Chicago Press, Chicago, 1954, pp. 601–661.
2. Forshufvud, S., Smith, H., and Wassen, A., Nature, 1961, 192, 103–105.
3. Smith, H., Forshufvud, S., and Wassen, A., Nature, 1962, 194, 725–726.
4. Giovanoli-Jakubczak, T., and Berg, G. G., Arch. Environ. Health, 1974, 28, 139–144.
5. Hammer, D. I., Finklea, J. F., Hendricks, R. H., Shy, C. M., and Horton, R. J. M., Amer. J. Epidem., 1971, 93, 84–92.
6. Ryabukhin, Y. S., J. Radioanal. Chem., 1980, 60, 7–30.
7. Lenihan, J. M. A., Smith, H., and Harvey, W., in *Nuclear Activation Techniques in the Life Sciences 1972*, Proceedings of a Symposium, Bled, International Atomic Energy Agency, Vienna, 10–14 April, 1972, pp. 195–212.
8. Chattopadhyay, A., Roberts, T. M., and Jervis, R. E., Arch. Environ. Health, 1977, 30, 226–236.
9. Strain, W. H., Steadman, L. T., Lankau, C. A., Berliner, W. P., and Pories, W. J., Lab. Clin. Med., 1966, 68, 244–249.
10. Klevay, L. M., Amer. J. Clin. Nutr., 1970, 23, 284–289.
11. Deeming, S. B., and Weber, C. W., Amer. J. Clin. Nutr., 1977, 30, 2047–2052.
12. Gershoff, S. N., McGandy, R. B., Nondasuta, A., Pisolyabutra, U., and Tantiwongse, P., Amer. J. Clin. Nutr., 1977, 30, 868–872.
13. Chittleborough, G., and Steel, B. J., Sci. Total Environ., 1980, 15, 25–35.
14. Mertz, W., Physiol. Rev., 1969, 49, 163–239.
15. Hambidge, K. M., Rodgerson, D. O., and O'Brien, D., Diabetes, 1968, 17, 517–519.
16. Benjanuvatra, N. K., and Bennion, M., Nutr. Rep. Internat., 1975, 12, 325–330.
17. Iyengar, G. V., Kollmer, W. E., and Bowen, H. M. J., *The Elemental Composition of Human Tissues and Body Fluids*, Verlag Chemie, Weinheim, 1978, p. 51.
18. Versieck, J., and Cornelius, R., Anal. Chim. Acta, 1980, 116, 217–254.
19. Katz, S. A., Amer. Lab., 1979, 11, 44–52.
20. anonymous, Chemistry, 1979, 52, 28–29.
21. Katz, S. A., and Wood, J. D., Chem. Internat., 1980, 6, 12–15.
22. Hambidge, K. M., Amer. J. Clin. Nutr., 1973, 26, 1212–1215.
23. Kopito, L. E., and Shwachman, H., J. Invest. Dermatol., 1975, 64, 342-348.
24. Valkovic, V., Rendic, D., and Phillips, G. C., Environ. Sci. Technol., 1975, 9, 1150–1152.
25. Valkovic, V., *Trace Elements in Hair*, Garland STPM Press, New York, 1977.
26. Anke, M., and Risch, M., *Haaranalyse und Spurenelementstatus*, Gustav Fischer Verlag, Jena, 1979.

27. Passwater, R. A., and Cranton, E. M., *Trace Elements, Hair Analysis, and Nutrition*, Keats Pub. Co., New Canaan, CT, 1983.
28. Valkovic, V., *Human Hair*, Vol. I & II, CRC Press, Boca Raton, FL, 1988.
29. The First Hair Symposium, Atlanta, 12–14 October, 1973.
30. The Second Hair Symposium, Atlanta, 13–15 October, 1978.
31. Second International Symposium: Trace Elements, Human Health, Hair Analysis, Amsterdam, 18–19 May, 1984.
32. Cranton, E. M., Bland, J. S., Chatt, A., Krakovitz, R., and Wright, J. V., J. Holist. Med., 1982, 4, 1–16.
33. Robbins, C. R., *Chemical and Physical Behavior of Human Hair*, Van Nostrand Reinhold Co., New York, 1979, p. 22.
34. Hopps, H. C., Sci. Total Environ., 1977, 7, 71–89.
35. Chittleborough, G., Sci. Total Environ., 1980, 14, 53–75.
36. Saitoh, M., Uzuka, M., and Sakamoto, M., J. Invest. Dermatol., 1970, 54, 65–81.
37. Rivlin, R. S., Amer. J. Med., 1983, 75, 489–493.
38. Airey, D., Sci. Total Environ., 1983, 31, 157–180.
39. Airey, D., Environ. Health Prospec., 1983, 52, 303–316.
40. Berg, D., and Kollmer, W. E., in *Trace Element Analytical Chemistry in Medicine and Biology*, Vol. 2, P. Bratter and P. Schramel, eds., Walter de Gruyter and Co., Berlin, 1983, pp. 571–583.
41. Hansen, J. C., Wulf, H. C., Kromann, N., and Aloge, K., Sci. Total Environ., 1983, 26, 233–243.
42. Kopito, L., Byers, R. K., and Shwachman, H., New England J. Med., 1967, 276, 949–953.
43. Kopito, L., Briley, A. M., and Shwachman, H., J. Amer. Med. Assoc., 1969, 209, 243–248.
44. Valentine, J. L., Kang, H. K., and Spivey, G., Environ. Res., 1979, 20, 24–32.
45. Yang, G., Wang, S., Zhou, R., and Sun, S., Amer. J. Clin. Nutr., 1983, 37, 872–881.
46. Klevay, L. M., Amer. J. Clin. Nutr., 1970, 23, 1194–1202.
47. Jacob, R. A., Klevay, L. M., and Logan, G. M., Amer. J. Clin. Nutr., 1978, 31, 477–480.
48. McKenzie, J. M., Amer. J. Clin. Nutr., 1979, 32, 570–579.
49. Bate, L. C., and Dyer, F. F., Nucleonics, 1965, 23, 74–81.
50. Bate, L. C., Internat. J. Appl. Radiat. Isotopes, 1966, 17, 417–423.
51. Gordus, A., J. Radioanal. Chem., 1973, 15, 229–243.
52. Toribara, T. Y., and Jackson, D. A., Clin. Chem., 1982, 28, 650–654.
53. Clanet, P., DeAntonio, S. M., Katz, S. A., and Scheiner, D. M., Clin. Chem., 1982, 28, 2450–2451.
54. Marzulli, F. N., and Brown, D. W. C., J. Soc. Cosmet. Chem., 1972, 23, 875–886.
55. Marzulli, F. N., Watlington, P. M., and Maibach, H. I., Curr. Prob. Dermatol., 1978, 7, 196–204.
56. Husain, M., Khaliquzzaman, M., Abdullah, M., Ahmed, I., and Khan, A. H., Internat. J. Appl. Radiat. Isotopes, 1980, 31, 527–533.
57. Briggs, M. H., Briggs, M., and Wakatama, A., Experientia, 1972, 15, 406–407.
58. Kapauan, P. A., Beltran, I. L., and Cruz, C. C., Philipp. J. Sci., 1982, 111, 145–155.
59. Takeuchi, T., Ann. Rep. Res. Reactor Inst. Kyoto Univ., 1978, 11, 177–185.
60. Qureshi, I. H., Chaudhary, M. S., and Ahmed, S., J. Radioanal. Chem., 1982, 68, 209–218.
61. Eads, E. A., and Lambdin, C. E., Environ. Res., 1973, 6, 247–252.
62. Schroeder, H. A., and Nason, A. P., J. Invest. Dermatol., 1968, 53, 71–78.
63. Turkstra, J., Beukes, P. J. L., Brits, R. J. N., and Hambleton-Jones, B. B., S. Afr. J. Sci., 1978, 74, 182–184.
64. Lech, J., Delles, F., and Culver, B., Varian Instr. Applic., 1974, 8, 8–9.
65. Varier, K. M., Nayak, A. K., and Mehta, G. K., IEEE Trans. Nucl. Sci., 1983, 30, 1316–1318.
66. Bos, A. J. J., Van Der Stap, C. C. A. H., Lenglet, W. J. M., Vis, R. D., and Valkovic, V., IEEE Trans. Nucl. Sci., 1983, 30, 1249–1251.
67. Laker, M., Lancet, 1982, July 31, 260–262.
68. Yurachek, J. P., Clemena, G. G., and Harrison, W. W., Anal. Chem., 1969, 41, 1666–1668.

69. Delves, H. T., Prog. Anal. Atomic Spectro., 1981, 4, 1–48.
70. Hilderbrand, D. C., and White, D. H., Clin. Chem., 1974, 20, 148–151.
71. Klevay, L. M., Arch. Intern. Med., 1978, 138, 1127–1128.
72. Bland, J., Orthomolec. Psych., 1980, 9, 24–32.
73. DeAntonio, S. M., Katz, S. A., Scheiner, D. M., and Wood, J. D., Clin. Chem., 1982, 28, 2411–2413.
74. Fergusson, J. E., Holzbecher, J., and Ryan, D. E., Sci. Total Environ., 1983, 26, 121–135.
75. Hinners, T. A., Terill, W. J., Kent, J. L., and Colucci, A. V., Environ. Health Prospec., 1974, 8, 191–199.
76. Weiss, D., Whitten, B., and Liddy, D., Science, 1972, 178, 69–70.
77. Flynn, A., Fratianne, R. B., Hill, C. A., Pories, W. J., and Strain, W. H., Amer. J. Clin. Nutr., 1971, 24, 893–894.
78. Rabinowitz, M., Wetherill, G., and Kopple, J., Arch. Environ. Health, 1976, 31, 220–223.
78a. Leyton, Can. Med. Assoc. J., 1985, 133, 1109.
79. Arunachalam, J., Gangadharon, S., and Yegnasubramanian, S., in *Nuclear Science Techniques in the Life Sciences 1978* IAEA-SM-227/24, International Atomic Energy Agency, Vienna, 1979, pp. 499–513.
80. Chittleborough, G., and Steel, B. J., Anal. Chim. Acta, 1980, 119, 235–241.
81. Orlando, P., Perdelli, F., Casadio, M., and Pecorari, D., Gioranle di Igiene Med. Preventiva, 1978, 18, 62–67.
82. Thatcher, R. W., Clin. Chem., 1983, 29, 461–462.
83. Dang, H. S., Jaiswal, D. D., Mehta, U., and Deshpande, A., Sci. Total Environ., 1983, 31, 187–192.
84. Rees, E. L., and Campbell, J., "Patterns of Trace Minerals in Hair and Relationships to Clinical States," Meeting, Academy of Orthomolecular Psychiatry, Detroit, May, 1974.
85. Sumie, Y., Tanaka, H., and Nishimura, M., Bull. Tokyo Med. Coll., 1982, 23, 15–24.
86. Lenihan, J. M. A., Smith, H., and Harvey, W., Brit. Dent. J., 1973, 135, 365–369.
87. Petering, H. G., Yeager, D. W., and Witherup, S. O., Arch. Environ. Health, 1971, 23, 202–207.
88. Takeuchi, T., Hayashi, T., Takada, J., Hayashi, Y., Koyama, M., Kozuka, H., Tsuji, H., Kusaka, Y., Ohmori, S., Shinogi, M., Aoki, A., Katayama, K., and Tomiyama, T., J. Radioanal. Chem., 1982, 70, 29–55.
89. Imahori, A., Fukushima, I., Shiobara, S., Yamagida, Y., and Tomura, K., J. Radioanal. Chem., 1979, 52, 167–180.
90. Reeves, R. D., Jolley, K. W., and Buckley, P. D., Bull. Environ. Contamin. Toxicol., 1975, 14, 579–587.
91. Creason, J. P., Hinners. T. A., Bumgarner, J. E., and Pinkerton, C., Clin. Chem., 1975, 21, 603–612.
92. Petering, H. G., Yeager, D. W., and Witherup, S. O., Arch. Environ. Health, 1973, 27, 327–330.
93. Hung, P. Q., Cholewa, M., Kajfosz, J., and Szymczyk, S., "PIXE Studies of Ethnic Differences of Trace and Other Elements Concentration in Human Hair," Proceedings of the 2nd International Workshop on Trace Element Analytical Chemistry in Medicine and Biology, Neuherberg, April, 1982.
94. Chen, S. Y., Collipp, P. J., Boasi, L. H., Isenschmid, D. S., Verolla, R. J., SanRoman, G. A., and Yeh, J. K., Ann. Nutr. Metab., 1982, 26, 186–190.
95. Moo, P. S., and Pillay, K. K. S., J. Radioanal. Chem., 1983, 77, 141–147.
96. Klevay, L. M., Arch. Environ. Health, 1973, 26, 169–172.
97. Wiesener, W., and Schaefer, U., Zentralbl. Pharm., Pharmakother. Laboratoriumsdiagn., 1982, 121, 459–463.
98. Katz, S. A., Bowen, H. M. J., Comaish, J. S., and Samitz, M. H., Brit. J. Dermatol., 1975, 92, 187–190.
99. Flesch, P., and Rothman, S., J. Invest. Dermatol., 1945, 6, 257–270.
100. Lerner, A. B., and Fitzpatrick, T. B., Physiol. Rev., 1950, 30, 91–126.
101. Dutcher, T. F., and Rothman, S., J. Invest. Dermatol., 1951, 17, 65–68.
102. Dorea, J. G., and Pereira, S. E., J. Nutr., 1983, 113, 2375–2381.

103. Sorenson, J. R. J., Levin, L. S., and Petering, H. G., Interface, 1973, 2, 17.
104. Jervis, R. E., Tiefenbach, B., and Chattopadhyay, A., J. Radioanal. Chem., 1977, 37, 751–760.
105. Baker, E. L., Hayes, C. G., Landrigen, P. J., Handke, J. L., Leger, R. T., Housworth, W. J., and Harrington, M., Amer. J. Epidem., 1977, 106, 261–273.
106. Obrusnik, I., and Bencko, V., Radiochem. Radioanal. Letters, 1979, 38, 186–195.
107. Lanzel, E., J. Radioanal. Chem., 1980, 58, 347–357.
108. Bhat, K. R., Arunachalam, J., Yegnasubramanian, S., and Gangedharan, S., Sci. Total Environ., 1982, 22, 169–178.
109. Clemente, G. F., Cigna-Rossi, L., and Santaroni, G. P., in *Nuclear Activation Techniques in the Life Sciences 1978,* International Atomic Energy Agency, Vienna, 1979, pp. 527–543.
110. Hunt, I. F., Murphy, N. J., Cleaver, A. E., Faraji, B., Swendseid, M. E., Coulson, A. H., Clark, V. A., Laine, N., Davis, C. J., and Smith, J. C., Amer. J. Clin. Nutr., 1983, 37, 572–582.
111. Lane, H. W., Warren, D. C., Squyres, N. S., and Cotham, A. C., Biol. Trace Element Res., 1982, 4, 83–93.
112. Greger, J. L., and Geissler, A. H., Amer. J. Clin. Nutr., 1978, 31, 633–637.
113. Reilly, C., Proc. Nutr. Soc. Australia, 1981, 6, 141–143.
114. Izumi, K., Tokyo Ika Daizaku Zasshi, 1983, 41, 43–49.
115. Deeming, S. B., and Weber, C. W., Amer. J. Clin. Nutr., 1978, 31, 1175–1180.
116. Klinger, G., Wiesener, W., and Dawcynski, H., Deutsch. Gesundheitswes., 1981, 36, 1740–1742.
117. Vir, S. C., and Lowe, A. H. G., Amer. J. Clin. Nutr.. 1981, 34, 1479–1483.
118. Kamel, H., Brown, D. H., Ottaway, J. M., and Smith, W. E., Talanta, 1977, 24, 309–313.
119. Williams, D. M., Atkins, C. L., Frens, D. B., and Bray, P. F., Pedi. Res., 1977, 11, 823–826.
119a.Doria, J. G., Costa, J. M. L., Holzbecher, J., Ryan, D. E., and Marsden, P. D., Clin. Chem., 1987, 33, 2081–2082.
120. Schroeder, H. A., *Trace Elements and Man,* Devin-Adair Co., Old Greenwich, CT, 1973, p. 31.
121. Hambidge, K. M., Hambidge, C., Jacobs, M., and Baum, J. D., Amer. J. Clin. Nutr., 1976, 29, 734–738.
122. Gibson, R. S., and DeWolfe, M. S., Pedi. Res., 1979, 13, 959–962.
123. Combs, D. K., Goodrich, R. D., and Meiske, J. C., J. Animal Sci., 1982, 54, 391–398.
124. Sanders, H. J., Chem. Eng. News, 1979, March 26, 27–48.
125. Faulkner, W. R., Lab. Mgmt, 1981, July, 21–35.
126. Olwin, J. H., J. Anal. Toxicol., 1977, 1, 245–251.
127. Schwartz, K., and Mertz, W., Arch. Biochem. Biophys., 1959, 85, 292–295.
128. Mertz, W., Fed. Proc., 1967, 26, 186–193.
129. Hart, E. B., Steinbock, H., Waddell, J., and Elevhjin. C. A., J. Biol. Chem., 1928, 77, 797–800.
130. Schwartz, K., and Milne, D. B., Bioinorganic Chem., 1972, 1, 355.
131. Messer, H. H., Wong, K., Wegner, M., Singer, L., and Armstrong, W. D., Nature, 1972, 240, 218–224.
132. Messer, H. H., Armstrong, W. D., and Singer, L., Science, 1972, 177, 893–896.
133. Maier, F. J., *Fluoridation,* CRC Press, Cleveland, 1972.
134. Chatin, A., C. R. Acad. Sci., 1852, 34, 14–16.
135. anonymous, *Recommended Dietary Allowances,* Food and Nutrition Board, National Research Council, Washington, 1974.
136. MacMunn, C. A., Phil. Trans. Royal Soc. London, 1886, 177, 267–271.
137. Skrede, S., and Seip, M., Scand. J. Hematol., 1979, 23, 232–238.
138. Ohira, Y., Edgerton, V. R., Gardner, G. W., and Senewiraine, B., J. Nutr. Sci. Vitaminol., 1980, 26, 375–379.
139. Jain, S. K., Yip, R., Pramanik, A. K., Dallman, P. R., and Shoket, S. B., J. Nutr., 1982, 112, 1230–1233.
140. Kemmerer, A. R., Elevhjin, C. A., and Hart, E. B., J. Biol. Chem., 1931, 92, 623–630.
141. Doisy, E. A., *Proceedings of the 6th Annual Conference on Trace Substances in Environmental Health,* D. D. Hempill, ed., University of Missouri Press, Columbia, 1973, p. 193.

142. Wenlock, R. W., Buss, D. H., and Dixon, E. J., Brit. J. Nutr., 1979, 41, 253-261.
143. anonymous, J. Amer. Med. Assoc., 1979, 241, 2051-2054.
144. Underwood, E. J., *Trace Elements in Human and Animal Nutrition, 3rd ed.*, Academic Press, New York, 1971.
145. Richard, D. A., and Westerfield, W. W., J. Biol. Chem., 1953, 203, 915-923.
146. Coughlan, M. P., J. Inherit. Metab. Dis., 1983, 6, 70.
147. Abumad, N. N., Schneider, A. J., and Steel, D., Amer. J. Clin. Nutr., 1981, 34, 2551-2254.
148. Fitzgerald, F. T., and Tierney, L. M., Adv. Intern. Med., 1984, 30, 337-358.
149. Nielsen, F. H., and Sandstead, H. H., Amer. J. Clin. Nutr., 1974, 27, 515-520.
150. Nielsen, F. H., and Ollerich, D. A., Fed. Proc., 1974, 33, 1767-1772.
151. anonymous, *Nickel*, National Academy of Sciences, Washington, 1975, pp. 82-85.
152. Sandstead, H. H., in *Nutrition in the 20th Century*, M. Winick, ed., John Wiley and Sons, Inc., New York, 1984, pp. 37-46.
152a. Iyengar, G. V., and Gopal-Ayengar, A. R., Ambio, 1988, 17, 31-35.
153. Baker, S. S., Lerman, R. H. and Krey, S. H., Amer. J. Clin. Nutr., 1983, 38, 769-772.
154. Carlisle, E. M., Science, 1972, 178, 619-623.
155. Schwartz. K., and Milne, D. B., Nature, 1972, 239, 333-334.
156. Schwartz, K., Milne, D. B., and Vinyard, E., Biochem. Biophys. Res. Communic., 1970, 40, 22-30.
157. Schwartz, K., Fed. Proc., 1974, 33, 1748-1756.
158. Hopkins, L. L., and Mohr, H. E., Fed. Proc., 1971, 30, 462.
159. Schwartz, K., and Milne, D. B., Science, 1971, 174, 426-427.
160. Todd, W. R., Elevhjin, C. A., and Hart, E. B., Amer. J. Physiol., 1934, 107, 146-155.
161. Sandstead, H. H., Prasad, A. S., and Schulert, A. R., Amer. J. Clin. Nutr., 1967, 20, 422-429.
162. Hambidge, K. M., Chaves, M. N., and Brown, R. M., Amer. J. Clin. Nutr., 1979, 32, 2532-2540.
163. Hambidge, K. M., Hambidge, C., Jacobs, M., and Balm, J. D., Pedi. Res., 1972, 6. 868-874.
164. Gershoff, S. N., McGandy, R. B., Nondasuta, A., Pisolyabutra, U., and Tantiwongse, P., Amer. J. Clin. Nutr., 1977, 30, 868-872.
165. McKenzie, J. M., Amer. J. Clin. Nutr., 1979, 32, 570-579.
166. Gibson, R. S., and DeWolfe, N. S., Nutr. Rep. Internat., 1980, 21, 341-349.
167. Gibson, R. S., J. Radioanal. Chem., 1982, 70, 175-189.
168. Dorea, J. G., Horner, M. R., Bezerra, V. L., Pereira, M. G., and Salomon, J. B., Human Nutr. Appl. Nutr.. 1982, 36A, 63-67.
169. Dorea, J. G., Alemida, I. S., Queiroz, E. F. O., and Horner, M. R., Ecol. Food Nutr., 1982, 12, 1-6.
170. Dorea, J. G., Amer. J. Clin. Nutr., 1981, 34, 2323-2324.
171. Kohrs, M. B., Choh, K. H., and Nordstrom, J. W., Nutr. Res., 1986, 6, 889-903.
172. Lines, D. R., and Bell, E. B., Proc. Nutr. Soc. New Zealand, 1977, 2, 31-37.
173. Ren, S., Wang, S., and Ye, G., Zhonghua Yufangyixue Zazhi, 1983, 17, 285-288.
174. Erten, J., Arcasoy A., Cavdar, A. O., and Cin, S., Amer. J. Clin. Nutr., 1978, 31, 1172-1174.
175. O'Leary, N. J., Mata, L. J., and Hegarty, P. V. J., Amer. J. Clin. Nutr., 1980, 33, 2194-2197.
176. Gentile, P. S., Trentalange, M. J., and Coleman, M., Pedi. Res., 1981, 15, 123-127.
177. Heinersdorff, N., and Taylor, T. G., Arch. Dis. Child., 1979, 54, 958-960.
178. Bradfield, R. B., Soohoo, T., and Baertl, J. M., Amer. J. Clin. Nutr., 1980, 33, 1315-1317.
179. Vivoli, G., Bergomi, M., Fantuzzi, G., Del Dot, M., Tonelli, E., Zanetti, F., and Gatto, M., Spurenelement Symposium V, Jena, DDR, July, 1986.
180. McDonald, L. D., Gibson, R. S., and Miles, J. E., Acta Pedi. Scand., 1982, 71, 785-789.
181. Higashi, A., Ikeda, T., Uehara, I., and Matsuda, I., Eup. J. Pedi., 1982, 138, 237-240.
182. Matsuda, I., Higashi, A., Ikeda, T., Uehara, I., and Koroki, Y., J. Pedi. Gastroenterol. Nutr., 1984, 3, 421-425.
183. Mahajan, S. K., Prasad, A. S., Rabban F., Briggs, W. A., and McDonald, F. D., Amer. J. Clin. Nutr., 1982, 36, 1177-1183.

184. Gupta, B. D., Dwarkanath P. K., and Miglani, N., Indian Pedi., 1978, 15, 825–825.
185. Chen, W., and Ren, S.. Kexue Tongboa, 1984, 29, 693–695.
186. Hambidge, K. M., Amer. J. Clin. Nutr., 1982, 36, 943–949.
186a. Barrett, S., J. Amer. Med. Assoc., 1985, 254, 1041–1045.
187. Gibson, R. S., Sci. Total Environ., 1984, 39, 93–101.
188. Bradfield, R. B., Corano, A., Baertl, J., and Graham G. G., Lancet, 1980, 11, 343–344.
189. Panday, V. K., Parameswaran, S. J., Raut, S. D., and DeCosta, H., Sci. Total Environ., 1983, 27, 261–264.
190. Machida, K., Matsubara, J., and Sugawara, K., Nutr. Rep. Internat., 1984, 29, 1145–1154.
191. Herber, R. F. M., Wibowo, A. A. E., Das, H. A., Egger, R. J., Van Deyck, W., and Ziehuis, R. L., Internat. Arch. Environ. Health, 1983, 53, 127–137.
192. Yang, G., Wang, G., Yin, T., Sun, S., Zhou, R., Man, R., Zhai, F., Guo, S., Wang, H., and You, D., Yingyang Xuebao, 1982, 4, 191–200.
193. Gallagher, M. L., Webb, P., Crounse, R., Bray, J., Webb, A., and Settle, E. A., Nutr. Res., 1984, 4, 577–582.
194. Xiashu, C., Guangoi, T., Junshi, C., Xuecun, C., Zhimei, W., and Keyou, G., Biol. Trace Element Res., 1980, 2, 91–93.
195. Clemente, G. F., Cigna-Rossi. L., and Santaroni, G. P., J. Radioanal. Chem., 1977, 37, 549–558.
196. Clemente, G. F., Cigna-Rossi, L., and Santaroni, G. P., in *Trace Elements in Environmental Health*, D. D. Hemphill, ed., University of Missouri Press, Columbia, 1978, pp. 23–30.
197. Kulachenko, V. P., S-kh. Biol., 1984, 7, 118–122.
198. Weider, B., and Hapgood, D., *The Murder of Napoleon*, Congdon and Lattes, Inc., New York, 1982.
199. Bowen, H. M. J., *Environmental Chemistry of the Elements*, Academic Press, New York, 1979, pp. 129–130.
200. Friberg, L.. Piscater, M., Nordberg, G., and Kjellstorm, T., *Cadmium in the Environment*, 2nd ed., CRC Press, Cleveland, 1974.
201. Horvath, D. J., in *Trace Substances and Health*, P. M. NewBerne, ed., Marcel Dekker, Inc., New York, 1976, pp. 340–341.
202. Bidstrup, L., *Toxicity of Mercury and Its Compounds*, Elsevier Publishing Co., Amsterdam, 1964, pp. 45–49.
203. Rabinowitz, M. B., Biol. Trace Element Res., 1987, 12, 223–229.
204. Canter, D. E., and Fernando, Q., J. Chem. Educ., 1979, 56, 490–495.
205. Taylor, A., and Marks, V., Anal. Clin. Biochem., 1977, 14, 297–300.
206. Kalman, S. M., Anal. Toxicol., 1977, 1, 277–281.
207. Campbell, B. C., and Baird, A. W., Brit. J. Intern. Med., 1977, 34, 298–304.
208. Gregus, Z., and Klaassen, C. D., Toxicol. Appl. Pharmacol., 1986, 85, 24–38.
209. Kollmer, W. E., and Berg, D., J. Radioanal. Chem., 1979, 52, 189–197.
210. Kollmer, W. E., J. Radioanal. Chem., 1980, 57, 535–541.
211. Kollmer, W. E., Sci. Total Environ., 1982, 25, 41–51.
212. Wesenberg, G., Fosse, G., Rasmussen, P., and Justesen, N. P. B., Internat. J. Environ. Stud., 1981, 16, 147–155.
213. Wesenberg, G. B. R., Internat. J. Environ. Stud., 1983, 20, 245–254.
214. Wesenberg, G. B. R., Internat. J. Environ. Stud., 1983, 30, 255–263.
215. Weigel, H. J., Jager, H. J., and Elmadfa, I., Arch. Environ. Contamin. Toxicol., 1984, 13, 279–287.
216. Ohmori, S., and Hashimoto, K., J. Radioanal. Nucl. Chem., 1985, 89, 277–285.
217. Scheiner, D. M., Katz, S. A., and Samitz, M. H., Environ. Res., 1976, 12, 355–357.
218. Yokel, R. A., Clin. Chem., 1982, 28, 662–665.
219. Hindmarsh, J. T., McLetchie, O. R., Heffernan, L. P. M., Hayne, O. A., Ellenberger, H. A., McCurdy, R. F., and Thiebaux, H. J., J. Anal. Toxicol., 1977, 1, 270–276.

220. Olguín, A., Jauge, P., Cebriàn, M., and Albores, A., Proc. West. Pharmacol. Soc., 1983, 26, 175–177.
221. Borgono, J., Vicent, P., Venturino, H., and Infarte, A., Environ. Health Prospect., 1977, 19, 103–105.
222. Horvath, A., Gig. Sanit., 1981, 6, 62–65.
223. Bozsai, G., Czegeny, I., and Karpati, Z., Kem. Lapja, 1984, 39, 121–123.
224. Bencko, V., and Symon, K., Environ. Res., 1977, 13, 378–385.
225. Morse, D. I., Harrington, J. M., Housworth, J., Landrigan, P. J., and Kelter, A., Clin. Toxicol., 1979, 14, 389–399.
226. Liu, C. T., Yan, K. L., Chen, Y., Ma, W. N., and Huang, C. K., Chong-hoa Yu Fang I Hsuch Tsa Chih, 1979, 13, 138.
227. Yamamura, Y., and Yamauchi, H., Indust. Health, 1980, 18, 203–210.
228. Feldman, R. G., Niles, C. A., Kelly-Nayes, M., Sax, D. S., Dixon, W. J., Thompson. D. J., and Landau, E., Neurology, 1979, 29, 939–944.
229. Gabor, S., Coldea, V., and Ossian, A., Spurenelement Symposium, Arsen, 3rd, Jena, 1980, pp. 283–286.
230. Pirl, J. N., Townsend, G. J., Valaitis, A. K., Grohlich, D., and Spikes, J. J., J. Anal. Toxicol., 1983, 7, 216–219.
231. Leslie, A. C. D., and Smith, H., Arch. Toxicol., 1978, 41, 163–167.
232. Lewin, P. K., and Hancock, R. G. V., Nature, 1982, 299, 627–628.
233. Grodzins, L., Trans. N. Y. Acad. Sci., 1980, 40, 93–98.
234. Kopito, L., Byers, R., and Shwachman, H., New England J. Med., 1967, 276, 949–953.
234a. Marzulli, F. N., and Maibach, H. I., Curr. Prob. Dermatol., 1978, 7, 196–204.
235. Niculescu, T., Dumitri, R., Botha, C.. Alexandrescu, R., and Manolescu, N., Brit. J. Indust. Med., 1983, 40, 67–70.
236. Clayton, E., and Wooller, K. K., IEEE Trans. on Nucl. Sci., 1983, 30, 1326–1328.
237. Sherlock, J. C., Lindsay, D. G., Hislop, J. E., Evans, W. H., and Collier, T. R.. Arch. Environ. Health, 1982, 37, 271–278.
238. Matthews, A. D., Environ. Res., 1983, 30, 305–312.
239. Brockhaus, A., Dolgner, R., Ewers, U., Kraemer, U., Soddemann, H., and Wiegand, H., Internat. Arch. Occup. Environ. Health, 1981, 48, 375–389.
240. Kijewski, H., Arch. Kriminol., 1984, 173, 36–44.
241. Metter, D., and Vock, R., Z. Rechtsmed., 1984, 91, 201–214.
242. Auld, D. S., in *Ultratrace Metal Analysis in Biological Sciences and Environment*, T. H. Risby, ed., Advances in Chemistry Series 172, American Chemical Society, Washington, 1979, p. 121.
243. Yunice, A. A., in *Ultratrace Metal Analysis in Biological Sciences and Environment*, T. H. Risby, ed., Advances in Chemistry Series 172, American Chemical Society, Washington, 1979, p. 233.
244. Maugh, T. H., Science, 1978, 202, 1271–1273.
245. Ritland, S., and Aaseth, J., Acta Pharmacol. Toxicol., 1986, 59, 195–201.
246. Cornelis, R., and Versieck, J., in *Treatise on Analytical Chemistry*, P. J. Elving, ed., John Wiley and Sons, Inc., New York, 1986, p. 671.
247. Kopito, L., Ellan, E., Shwachman, H., and Rossen, E., Pediatrics, 1972, 49, 620–624.
248. Stebbing, J. B., Turner, M. O., and Franz, K. B., Magnesium Bull., 1982, 4, 131–134.
249. Rudolph, C. S., J. Internat. Acad. Prev. Med., 1977, June, 1–23.
250. Martin, G. M., Nature, 1964, 202, 903–904.
251. Lott, I. T., DiPaolo, R., Schwartz, D., Janowska, S., and Kanter, J. M., New England J. Med., 1975, 292, 197–199.
252. Williams, D. M., Atkins, C. L., Frens, D. B., and Bray, P. F., Pedi. Res., 1977, 11, 823–826.
253. Okada, K., and Myiao, M., Acta Paediatrica Japonica, 1982, 24, 460–466.
254. Spruit, D., and Bongaarts, P. J. M., in *Clinical Chemistry and Chemical Toxicology of Metals*, S. S. Brown, ed., Elsevier, Amsterdam, 1977, pp. 261–264.
255. Mertz, W., Clin. Chem., 1975, 21, 468–475.

256. Hambidge, K. M., and Rodgerson, D. O., Amer. J. Obstet. Gynecol., 1969, 103, 320–321.
257. Rosson, J. W., Foster, K. J., Watton, R. I., Monro, P. P., Taylor, T. G., and Albert, K. G. M. M., Clin. Chim. Acta, 1979, 93, 299–304.
258. Rabinowitz, M. B., Levin, S. R., and Gonick, H. C., Metab. Clin. Exper., 1980, 29, 355–364.
259. Hunt, A. E., *Effect of Chromium Supplementation on Hair Chromium Concentration and Diabetic Status*, Diss. Abstr. Internat. B., 1984, 44, 2383.
260. Addink, N. W., and Frank, L. J., Nature, 1962, 193, 1190.
261. Lin, H., Chan, W., and Fang, Y., Nutr. Rep. Internat., 1977, 15, 635–643.
262. Zheng, S., We, H., Luo, X. Hu, G., and Shang, A., Zhonghua Zhongliu Zozhi, 1982, 4, 174–177.
262a. Zeng, X., Yao, H., Mu, M., Yang, J., Wang, Z., Chang, H., and Ye, Y., Nucl. Inst. Methods Phys. Res., 1987, B22, 172–175.
263. Wiesener, W., Gorner, W., Niese, S., Baldauf, K., Grund, W., Hennig, M., and Mende, T., Isotopenpraxis, 1981, 17, 278–282.
264. Wiesener, W., Gorner, W., and Niese, S., in *Nuclear Activation Techniques in the Life Sciences 1978*, International Atomic Energy Agency, Vienna, 1979, pp. 307–320.
265. Mende, T., Wiesener, W., Franke, W. G., Domschke, S., and Gorner, W., Isotopenpraxis, 1984, 20, 301–303.
265a. Kwiatek, W. M., Cholewa, M., Jones, K. W., Shore, R. E., and Redrick, A. L., Nucl. Inst. Methods Phys. Res., 1987, B22, 166–171.
265b. Janicki, K., Dobrowolski, J., and Krasnicki, K., Chemosphere, 1987, 16, 253–257.
266. Thimaya, S., and Ganapathy, S. N., Sci. Total Environ., 1982, 24, 41–49.
267. Terai, M., Akabane, A., Ohno, K., Sakurai, S., Tsunoda, F., Hashimoto, K., and Nishida, G., J. Radioanal. Chem., 1979, 52, 143–152.
268. Ying, T., Sun, S., Wang, H., You, T., and Yang, K., Ching-hua Yu I Hsuch Tsa Chih, 1979, 13, 207–210.
269. Hsu, K., Hsueh, W., Chang, P., Fung, T., Hung, S., and Liang, W., Chang-hsi Hsin I Yao, 1980, 9, 43–46.
270. Yang, G., Wang, G., Yin, T., Sun, S., Zhou, R., Man, R., Zhai F., Gou, S., Wang, H., and You, D., Yingyang Xuebao, 1983, 5, 191–200.
271. Jiang, X., An, R., Wei, P., Zhang, G., and Lina, X., Baichiuen Yike Xeubao, 1982, 8, 12–17.
272. Li, J., and Chen, D., Haunjing Kexue, 1981, 2, 338–341.
273. Li, J., Ren, S., and Chen, D., Haunjing Kexue, 1982, 3, 91–101.
274. Hou, S., and Zhu, Z., Haunjing Kexue, 1982, 3, 18–23.
275. Wang, M., Yingyang Xuebao, 1982, 4, 201–207.
276. Yang, G., Zhou, R., Sun, S., Wang, S., and Li, S., Yingyang Xuebao, 1982, 4, 81–89.
277. Bacso, J., Kovacs, P., and Horvath, S., Radiochem. Radioanal. Letters, 1978, 33, 273–280.
278. Bacso, J., Horvath, M., Horvath, S., Baliczky, T., Mahunka, I., and Szucs, M., Magyar Belorvosi Archivum, 1982, 35, 245–250.
279. Bacso, J., Sarkadi, L., and Koltay, E., Internat. J. Appl. Radiat. Isotopes, 1982, 33, 5–11.
280. Bacso, J., J. Radioanal. Nucl. Chem., 1984, 83, 167–173.
281. Bacso, J., Lusztig, G., Pal, A., and Uzonyi, I., Exper. Pathol., 1986, 29, 119–125.
282. Bacso, J., Uzonyi, I., and Katz, S. A., Biol. Trace Element Res., 1987, 12, 383–387.
283. Saltman, P., Ann. Intern. Med., 1983, 98, 823–827.
284. Whanger, P. D., Environ. Health Prospec., 1979, 28, 151–171.
285. Medeiros, D., and Borgman, R., Bull. Environ. Contamin. Toxicol., 29, 190–195.
286. Medeiros, D., and Borgman, R., Nutr. Res., 1982, 2, 455–466.
287. Medeiros, D., Pellum, L., and Brown, B., Nutr. Res., 1983, 3, 51–60.
288. Medeiros, D., and Pellum, L., Bull. Environ. Contamin. Toxicol., 1985, 34, 163–169.
289. Chen, X., Wang, Y., and Qin, J., Nanjing Dawue Xuebao Ziran Kexue, 1983, 4, 661–670.
290. Tsukamoto, Y., Iwanami, S., and Marumo, F., Kyoto Daigaku Genshiro Jikkensho, 1981, KUR-RI-TR-206, 1–6.

291. Mahajan, S. K., Prasad, A. S., Rabbani, P., Briggs, W. A., and McDonald, F. D., Amer. J. Clin. Nutr., 1982, 36, 1177-1183.
292. Tomza, U., and Maenhaut, W., J. Radioanal. Nucl. Chem., 1984, 86, 209-220.
293. DeGroot, H. J., DeHaas, E. J. M., D'Haese, P., Heyndrickx, A., and DeWolff, F. A., Pharm. Weekb., 1984, 6, 11-15.
294. Marumo, F., Tsukomoto, Y., Iwanami, S., Kishimoto, T., and Yamagami, S., Nephron, 1984, 38, 267-272.
295. Lenihan, J., in *Measuring and Monitoring the Environment*, J. Lenihan and W. W. Fletcher, eds., Academic Press, New York, 1978, pp. 66-86.
296. The Clean Air Act, public law 83-206.
297. The Clear Water Act, public law 92-500.
298. The Occupational Health and Safety Act, public law 93-523.
299. Lenihan, J. M. A., Smith, H., and Harvey, W., Brit. J. Dent., 1973, 107, 803-811.
300. Lin, S. M., Chiang, C. H., Tseng, C. L., and Yang, M. H., Radiochem. Radioanal. Letters, 1982, 56, 261-272.
301. Lee, T. S., and Sohn, D. H., Yakhak Hoe Chi, 1979, 23, 17-29.
302. Yatim, S., and Samsudin, U., Majalah Batan, 1984, 3, 23-31.
303. Francis, P. C., Birge, W. J., Roberts, B. J., and Block, J. A., J. Toxicol. Environ. Health, 1982, 10, 667-672.
304. Yamanaka, S., Tanaka, H., and Mishimura, M., Bull. Tokyo Dent. Coll., 1982, 23, 15-24.
305. McMullin, J. F., Pritchard, J. G., and Sikondari, A. H., Analyst, 1982, 107, 803-814.
306. Pritchard, J. G., McMullin, J. F., and Sikondari, A. H., Brit. J. Dent., 1982, 153, 333-336.
307. Muszynska-Zimma, E., Polski Tygodnik Lekarski, 1981, 36, 1195-1197.
308. Tartakovkaya, L. Y., Bykov, N. A., and Gridin, N. M., Fig. Tr. Prof. Zabol., 1979, 8, 41-42.
309. Akashi, J., Fukushima, I., and Imahori, A., J. Radioanal. Chem., 1982, 68, 59-65.
310. Raghupathy, L., and Sharma, V. N., Sci. Total Environ., 1985, 41, 73-78.
311. Tomza, U., Janicki, T., and Kosman, J., Spurenelement Symposium IV, Leipzig, 1983, pp. 362-368.
312. Tomza, U., Janicki, T., and Kosman, J., Radiochem. Radioanal. Letters, 1983, 58, 209-220.
313. Finelli, V. N., Boscolo, P., Salimei, E., Messineo, A., and Carelli, G., Proceedings of the 3rd International Conference on Heavy Metals in the Environment, Edinburgh, 1981, pp. 475-478.
314. Ohmori, S., J. Radioanal. Nucl. Chem., 1984, 84, 451-459.
314a. Jamall, I. S.. and Jaffer, R. A., Bull. Environ. Contam. Toxicol., 1987, 39, 608-614.
315. Naranjit, D., Thomassen, Y., Van Loon, J. C., Anal. Chim. Acta, 1979, 110, 307-312.
316. Zatka, V. J., Amer. Indust. Hyg. Assoc. J., 1985, 46, 327-331.
317. Bergert, K. D., Voigt, H., and Holler, U., Z. Gesamte Inn. Med. Ihre Grenzgeb., 1982, 37, 504-507.
318. Wiesener, W., and Grund, W., Isotopenpraxis, 1978, 14, 147-148.
319. Grund, W., Zlv. Mitt., 1979, 21, 630-636.
320. Grund, W., Schneider, W. D., and Wiesener, W., J. Radioanal. Chem., 1980, 58, 319-326.
321. Liebich, R. Schneider, W. D., and Wiesener, W., Zentralbl. Pharm. Pharmakother. Laboratoriumsdiagn., 1982, 121, 471-474.
322. Ellis, K. J., Yasumura, S., and Cohn, S. H., Amer. J. Indust. Med., 1981, 2, 32-33.
323. Ellis, K. J., Yasumura, S., Vartsky, D., and Cohn, S. H., Fundam. Appl. Toxicol., 1983, 3, 167-174.
324. Anke, M., Gruen, M., Kronemann, H., Schneider, H. J., Wiss. Z. Karl Marx Univ., 1980, 29, 515-522.
325. Brueckner, C., and Linsel, K., Kadmium Symposium 1977, Jena, 1977, pp. 312-316.
326. Cagnett, P., Cigna-Rossi, L., Clemente, G. F., and Santaroni, G. P., Commission of the European Communities Report EUR 5360, 1975, pp. 1451-1460.
327. Wiadrowska, B., and Syrowatka, T., Rocz. Panstw. Zakl. Hig., 1983, 34, 87-94.

328. Torres, P. J., Gomez-Gonzales, J. A., and Alvarez, G. P., Ber. Internat. Kolloq. Verhuetung Arbeitsumfallen Berufskr. Chem. Ind., 8th., 1982, Berlin, pp. 449–480.
329. Opekar, B., Hruska, J., and Bude, O., Prac. Lek., 1979, 31, 226–230.
330. Dubinskaya, N. A., Latv. P. S. R. Zinat. Akad. Vestis, 1980, 2, 16–22.
331. Bencko, V., Erben, K., Zmatlikova, K., Filkova, L., and Tichy, M., Csek. Hyg., 1982, 27, 206–211.
332. Fergusson, J. E., Hibbard, K. A., and Ting, R. L. H., Environ. Pollut., 1981, 2, 235–248.
333. Weber, C. W., Nelson, G. W., de Vaquera, M. V., and Pearson, P. B., Nutr. Rep. Internat., 1984, 30, 1009–1018.
333a. Burguera, J. L., Burgeura, M., Rondon, C. E., Rivas, C., Burguera, J. A., and Alarcon, J., Trace Elements Electrolytes Health Dis., 1987, 1, 21–26.
334. Dumitru, R., Niculescu, T., and Botha, C., Rev. Ig., Bacteriol., Virusol., Parazitol., Epidemiol., 1982, 31, 227–234.
335. Grandjean, P., Devel. Toxicol. Environ. Sci., 1987, 4, 311–318.
336. Ndiokwere, Ch. L., Environ. Pollut., 1985, 9, 95–105.
337. Bertram, H. P., Kemper, F. H., Muller, C., and Cuellar, J. A., personal communication, 1986.
338. Gabor, S., Coldea, V., and Modercea, M., Rev. Ig. Bacteriol., Virusol., Parazitol., Epidemiol., Pneumoffiziol., 1978, 27, 335–339.
339. Saner, G., Yuzbasiyan, V., and Cigdem, S., Brit. J. Indust. Med., 1984, 41, 263–266.
340. Wrzeniowska, K., Cempel, M., and Byczkowski, S., Bromatol. Chem. Toksyol., 1979, 12, 229–233.
341. Paciga, J. J., Chattopadhyay, A., and Jervis, R. E., Proceedings of the 2nd International Conference on Nuclear Methods in Environmental Research, 1974, pp. 286–300.
342. Sonneborn, M., BGA-Ber., 1978, 1, 103–107.
343. Milosevic, M., Petrovic, L., Petrovic, D., and Pejuskovic, B., Arh. Hig. Rada Toksikol., 1980, 31, 209–217.
344. Nemenko, B. A., and Goncharov, N. P., Zdravookhr. Kaz., 1983, 8, 35–37.
345. Hartwell, T. D., Handy, R. W., Harris, B. S., Williams, S. R., and Gehlbach, Arch. Environ. Health, 1983, 38, 284–295.
346. Wibowo, A. A. E., Brunekreek, B., Lebret, E., and Pieters, H., Internat. Arch. Occup. Environ. Health, 1980, 46, 275–280.
347. Jervis, R. E., and Tiefenbach, B., in *Nuclear Activation Techniques in the Life Sciences 1978*, International Atomic Energy Agency, Vienna, 1978, pp. 627–642.
348. Mitoma, S., Sato, M., Tachibara, T., Fujino, T., Miyazaki, T., Fujii, M., and Ikebe, H., Kyushu Yakugakkai Kaiho, 1976, 30, 147–152.
349. Ghelberg, N. W., and Bodor, E., International Conference, Management and Control of Heavy Metals in the Environment, 1979, pp. 163–166.
350. Ghelberg, N. W., Bodor, E., and Piersica, Z., International Meeting of the Israeli Ecology Society, 1983, pp. 577–584.
351. Bencko, V., Arbetova, D., Skupenova, V., and Papayova, A., Proceedings of the International Conference, Industrial and Environmental Xenobiotics, 1980, pp. 69–70.
352. Houtman, J. P. W., de Bruin, M., and de Goeij, J. J., in *Nuclear Activation Techniques in the Life Sciences 1978*, International Atomic Energy Agency, Vienna, 1979, pp. 599–614.
353. Auermann, E., Seidler, G., and Kneuer, M., Nahrung, 1977, 21, 799–806.
354. Obrusnik, I., Starkova, B., Blazek, V., and Bencko, V., J. Radioanal. Chem., 1979, 54, 311–324.
355. Johannesson, T., Lunde, G., and Steinnes, E., Acta Pharmacol. Toxicol., 1981, 48, 185–189.
356. Folio, M. R., Hennigan, C., and Errera, J., Environ. Pollut., 1982, 29, 261–269.
357. Kapauan, P. A., *Neutron Activation Analysis of Hair in Relation to Geographical Location and Extent of Industrialization*, Report IAEA R 2139 F, International Atomic Energy Agency, Vienna, 1981.
358. Kapauan, P., Beltran, I., and Cruz, C., Phillippine J. Sci., 1982, 111, 145–155.
359. Lee, Y. J., and Cha, C. W., Koryo Taehai Uikwa Taehak Chapchi, 1979, 16, 83–90.

360. Kim, N. B., *Trace Element Analysis of Human Hair by Neutron Activation Technique,* Report IAEA R 2535 F, International Atomic Energy Agency, Vienna, 1982.
361. Watanabe, H., Matsushita, S., Ogawa, T., Murayama, H., and Nagakura, E., Hyogo Ken Eisei Kenkyusho Kenkyu Hokoku, 1974, 9, 1–8.
362. Imahori, A., Fukushima, I., Shiobara, S., Yanagida, T., and Tomura, K., J. Radioanal. Chem., 1979, 52, 167–180.
363. Dissayayake, C. B., Senaratne, A., and Weerasooriya, S. V. R., Internat. J. Environ. Studies, 1984, 23, 41–48.
364. Lux, J., and Rauh, W., Pedagog. Naturwiss. Chem., 1982, 1, 24–25.
365. Caccuri, S., Decora, L., and Rossi, A., *Lead Content of Hair as an Index of Ambient Exposure and Poisoning,* CEC Report EUR 5360, Commission of the European Communities, Brussels, 1975.
366. Gruen, M., Anke, M., Hennig, A., and Kronemann, H., "Lead Content of Hair and Wool as an Indicator of Lead Burden," Spurelement Symposium, IV, Leipzig 1983.
367. Engst, R., Lauterbach, K., Kronig, R., and Beckmann, G., Nahrung, 1983, 27, 147–163.
368. Mankovska, B., Biologia (Bratislava), 1980, 35, 547–551.
369. Malenchenko, A., *Concentrations of Natural Radionuclides and Certain Toxic Trace Elements in Hair of Persons Living in Industrial and Agricultural Areas of Byelorussia,* Report IAEA R 2659 F, International Atomic Energy Agency, Vienna, 1983.
370. Golubenkov, A. M., and Malenchenko, A. F., Gig. Sanit., 1984, 7, 33–35.
371. Muszynska-Zimna, E., Bromatol. Chem. Toksykol., 1982, 15, 127–128.
372. Szuck, B., and Kurys, H., Rocz. Panstw. Zakl. Hig., 1982, 33, 143–148.
373. Dutkiewicz, T., Kulka, E., Sokolowska, D., and Woyciechowska, E., Rocz. Panstw. Zakl. Hig., 1978, 29, 299–301.
374. Dutkiewicz, T., Paprotny, W., Sokolowska, D., Kulka, E., Woyciechowska, E., Dybczynski, R., and Sterlinski, S., Chem. Anal., 1978, 23, 261–272.
375. Skorkowska-Zieleniewska, J., Symonowicz, H., and Marszal, P., Rocz. Panstw. Zakl. Hig., 1983, 34, 175–179.
376. Ahmed, M., "Study of Lead Pollution in School Children in Saudi Arabia," 2nd Report of Research Projects Sponsored by SANCST at the King Abdulaziz University, 1987.
377. Southwick, J. W., Western, A. E., Beck, M. N., Whitley, T., Isaacs, R., Petajan, J., and Hansen, C. D., in *Arsenic: Industrial, Biomedical, and Environmental Prospectives,* W. H. Lederer and R. J. Fensterheim, eds., Van Nostrand Reinhold, New York, 1983, pp. 210–225.
378. Cortes, E., Cassorla, V., Munoz, L., Gras, N., and Krishnan, S. S., Radiochem. Radioanal. Letters, 1981, 50, 177–184.
379. Valentine, J. L., Kang, H. K., Dang, P. M., and Schluchter, M., J. Toxicol. Environ. Health, 1980, 6, 731–736.
380. Valentine, J. L., Kang, H. K., Dang, P. M., and Spivey, G., in *Selenium in Biology and Medicine,* Spaliholz, J. E., Martin, J. L., and Ganther, A. E., eds., Avi, Westport, CT, 1981, pp. 354–357.
381. Cigna-Rossi, L., Clemente, G. F., and Santaroni, G., *Mercury and Selenium Distribution in a Defined Area and in Its Population,* Commission on National Nuclear Energy Report RT/PROT[16]29, 1976.
382. Uyeta, M., Chickasawa, K., and Mazaki, M., Shokuhin Eiseigaku Zashi, 1978, 19, 105–111.
383. Riolfatti, M., Ig. Mod., 1977, 70, 170–187.
384. Gras, G., and Mondain, J., Rev. Internat. Oceanographic Med., 1980, 59, 63–70.
385. Lin, H., Hunajing Kexue, 1983, 3, 65–68.
386. Sivalingam, P. M., and Sani, A. B., Marine Pollut. Bull., 1980, 11, 188–191.
387. Suckcharoen, S., Nuorteva, P., and Hasaen, E., Ambio, 1978, 7, 113–116.
388. Kyle, J. H., and Ghani, N., Arch. Environ. Health, 1982, 37, 266–271.
389. Kyle, J. H., and Ghani, N., Sci. Total Environ., 1983, 26, 157–162.
390. Nishima, T., Ikeda, S., Tada, T., Yagyu, H., and Mizoguchi, I., Tokyo Toritsu Eisei Kenkyusho Kenkyu Nempo, 1976, 27, 258–263.

391. Suzuki, T., Shishido-Kashiwazaki, S., Igata, A., and Niina, K., Ecol. Food Nutr., 1979, 8, 117–122.
392. Kitasono, M., and Yamamoto, M., Kogoshima-ken Kogai Eisei Kenkyusho Ho, 1980, 16, 74–92.
393. Sakurai, M., Nippon Koshu Eisei Zasshi, 1984, 31, 577–584.
393a. Tsugane, S., and Kondo, H., Sci. Total Environ., 1987, 63, 69–76.
394. Ferreiro, M., Danier, B., DeSouza, S., and Boas, A., Cienc. Cult., 1980, 32, 89–95.
395. Phelps, R. W., Clarkson, T. W., Kershaw, T. G., and Wheatley, B., Arch. Environ. Health, 1980, 35, 161–168.
396. Harada, M., Fujino, T., Akagi, T., and Nishigaki, S., Kumamoto Med. J., 1977, 30, 57–64.
397. Haxton, J., Lindsay, D. G., Hislop, J. S., Salmon, L., Dixon, E. J., Evans, W. H., Reid, J. R., Hewitt, C. J., and Jeffries, D. F., Environ. Res., 1979, 18, 351–368.
398. Hislop, J. S., Collier, T. R., White, G. P., Khathing, D. T., and French, E., *Proceedings of the Second International Conference on Chemical Toxicology and Clinical Chemistry*, S. S. Brown and J. Savoy, eds., Academic Press, London, 1983, pp. 145–148.
399. Den Tunkelaar, E. M., Van Esch, G. H., Hofman, B., Schuller, P. L., and Zwiers, J. H. L., *Mercury and Other Elements in Blood of the Dutch Population*, Commission of the European Communities Report EUR 5360, 1974.
400. Lodenius, M., and Seppanen, A., Chemosphere, 1982, 11, 755–759.
401. Lodenius, M., Seppanen, A., and Herranen, M., Water, Air, Soil Pollut., 1983, 19, 237–246.
402. Matsubara, J., and Machida, K., Environ. Res., 1985, 38, 225–238.
403. Limic, N., and Valkovic, V., Bull. Environ. Contamin. Toxicol., 1986, 37, 925–930.
404. Seta, S., Sato, M., Yoshino, M., and Miyasaka, S., Scanning Electron Microscopy, 1982, 1, 127–140.
405. Toribara, T. Y., Jackson, D. A., and French, W. R., Anal. Chem., 1982, 54, 1844–1849.
406. Hong-Kou, L., Malmqvist, K. G., Carlsson, L. E., and Akselsson, K. R., Nucl. Instr. Methods Phys. Res., 1984, B3, 347–351.
407. Orlic, I., Makjanic, J., and Valkovic, V., Nucl. Instr. Methods Phys. Res., 1984, 3, 250–252.
408. Bos, A. J. J., Van Der Stap, C. C. A. H., Valkovic, V., Vis, R. D., and Verheul, H., Nucl. Instr. Methods Phys. Res., 1984, 3, 654–659.
409. Ryabukhin, Y. S., *Activation Analysis of Hair as an Indicator of Contamination of Man by Environmental Pollutants*, IAEA Report IAEA/RL/50, International Atomic Energy Agency, Vienna, October, 1978.
410. M'Baku, S. B., "Invitation to Participate in an IAEA Co-ordinated Research Programme," International Atomic Energy Agency, Vienna, June, 1983.
410a. Friel, J. K., and Ngyuen, C. D., Clin. Chem., 1986, 32, 739–742.
411. Cornelius, R., and Speecke, A., Forensic Sci. Soc. J., 1971, 11, 29–46.
411a. Rakovic, M., and Pilecka, N., J. Radioanal. Nucl. Chem. Letters, 1987, 119, 61–65.
411b. Pilecka, N., Rakovic, M., and Obrusnik, J. Radioanal. Nucl. Chem. Letters, 1987, 118, 277–282.
412. Assarian, G. S., and Oberleas, D., Clin. Chem., 1977, 23, 1717–1772.
413. Ryan, D. E., Holzbecher, J., and Stuart, C. D., Clin. Chem., 1978, 24, 1996–2000.
414. Salmela, S., Vuori. E., and Kilpio, J. O., Anal. Chim. Acta, 1981, 125, 131–137.
415. Kumpulainen, J., Salmela, S., Vuori, E., and Lehto, J., Anal. Chim. Acta, 1982, 138, 361–364.
416. Mattera, V. D., Arbige, V. A., Tomellini, S. A., Erbe, D. A., Doxtader, M. M., and Forcè, R. K., Anal. Chim. Acta, 1981, 124, 409–414.
417. Kollmer, W. E., Sci. Total Environ., 1983, 27, 251–259.
418. Chatt, A., Sajjad, M., DeSilva, K. N., and Secord, C. A., *Health-Related Monitoring of Trace Element Pollutants Using Nuclear Techniques*, IAEA-TECDOC-330, International Atomic Energy Agency, Vienna, 1985, pp. 33–49.
419. Suzuki, T., Hongo, T., Morita, M., and Yamamoto, R., Sci. Total Environ., 1984, 39, 81–91.
420. Buckley, R. A., and Dreosti, I., Amer. J. Clin. Nutr., 1984, 40, 840–846.
421. Thiery, M., Heyndrickx, A., and Uyttersprot, C., IRCS Med. Sci., 1984, 12, 247.
422. Das, H. A., Dejkumhang, M. M., Herber, R. F. M., Hoede, D., and van der Sloot, H. A.,

Instrumental Neutron Activation Analysis of Human Hair and Related Radiotracer Experiments on Washing and Leaching, Report ECN-107, Netherlands Energy Research Foundation, Petten, 1981.
423. Pankhurst, C. A., and Pate, B. D., Rev. Anal. Chem., 1979, 4, 111–235.
424. Czauderna, M., J. Radioanal. Nucl. Chem., 1985, 89, 13–22.
425. Biso, J. N., Cohen, I. M., and Resnizky, S. M., Radiochem. Radioanal. Letters, 1983, 58, 175–180.
426. Pritchard, J. G., and Saied, S. O. Analysi, 1986, 111, 29–35.
427. Das, H. A., Hoede, D., Nieuwendijk, B. J. T., van der Sloot, H. A., Teunissen, G. J. A., and Woittiez, J. R. W., *Determination of Arsenic, Selenium, and Antimony by Neutron Activation Analysis. Application to Hair Samples*, Report ECN-131, Netherlands Energy Research Foundation, Petten, April, 1983.
428. Bayat, I., Moattar, F., and Kazamei, H., "Determination of Arsenic in Human Hair by Destructive Neutron Activation Analysis," Conference on Analytical Chemistry in Nuclear Technology, Karlsruhe, 1985.
429. Harrison, W. W., Yurachek, J. P., and Benson, C. A., Clin. Chim. Acta, 1969, 23. 83–91.
430. Nechay, M. W., and Sunderman, F. W., Anal. Clin. Lab. Sci., 1973, 3, 30–35.
431. Salgado, P. E. T., Larini, L., and Santos, A. C., Rev. Cienc. Farm., 1983, 5, 167–170.
432. Bagliano, G., Benischek, F., and Huber, I., Anal. Chim. Acta, 1981, 123, 45–56.
433. Voellkopf, U., and Grobenski, Z., Atomic Spectro., 1984, 5, 115–122.
434. Guillard, O., Brugler, J-C., Piriou, A., Ménard, M., Gombert, J., and Reiss, D., Clin. Chem., 1984, 30, 1642–1645.
435. Nord, P. J., Kadaba, M. P., and Sorenson, J. R. J.. Arch. Environ. Health, 1973, 27, 40–44.
436. Peter, F., and Strunc, G., Clin. Chem., 1984, 30, 893–895.
437. Suzuki, T., and Yamamoto, R., Bull. Environ. Contamin. Toxicol., 1982, 28, 186–188.
438. Greenwood, M. R., Dhahir, P., Clarkson, T. W., Farant, J. P., Chartrand, A., and Khayat, A., J. Anal. Toxicol., 1977, 1, 265–269.
439. Sakashita, H., Oda, S., and Kamada, H., Bunko Kenkyu, 1979, 28, 140–144.
440. Dermelj, M., Horvat, M., Byrne, A. R., and Stegnar, P., Chemosphere, 1987, 16, 877–886.
441. Clayton, E., Chapman, J. F., and Wooller, K. K., IEEE Trans. Nucl. Sci., 1983, 30, 1323–1325.
442. Badica, T., Ciortea, C., Cojocaru, M., Ivascu, M., Popa, A., Petrovici, A., Popescu, I., Salagean, M., and Spiridon, S., Nucl. Instr. Methods Phys. Res., 1984, B3, 288–290.
443. Baptista, G. B., Montenegro. E. C., Paschoa, A. S., and Barros Leite, C. V., Nucl. Instr. Methods, 1981, 181, 263–267.
444. Pillay, A. E., and Peisach M., J. Radioanal. Chem., 1981, 63, 85–95.
445. Whitehead, N. E., Nucl. Instr. Methods, 1979, 164, 381–383.
446. Mahrok, M. F., Crumpton, D., and Francois, P. E., Nucl. Instr. Methods Phys. Res., 1984, B4, 120–126.
447. Hall, G. S., Roach, N., Simmons, U., Cong, H.. Lee, M-I, and Cummings, E., J. Radioanal. Nucl. Chem., 1984, 82, 329–339.
448. Paschoa, A. S., Baptista, G. B., Mauricio. G. M., Barros Leite, C. V., Lerner, Y. B., and Issler, P. F., Nucl. Instr. Methods Phys. Res. B3, 1984, 352–356.
449. Henley, E. C., Kassouny, M. E., Nelson, J. W., Science, 1977, 197, 277–278.
450. Vis, R. D., Bos, A. J. J., Ullings, F., Houtman, J. P. W., and Verheul, H., Nucl. Instr. Methods, 1982, authors' proof.
451. Christensen, L. H., Ugeskr. Laeg., 1980, 142, 10–12.
452. Wang, J., Hejishu, 1987, 10, 14–16.
453. Monasterios, C. V., Jones, A. M., and Salin, E. D., Anal. Chem., 1986, 58, 780–785.
454. Chaudhri, M. A., Biol. Trace Element Res., 1987, 13, 417–421.
455. Zhao, C., Shifam Daxue Xuebao Ziran Kexueban, 1987, 2, 61–66.
456. Marquardt, D., Z. Erke. Atmungs-organe, 1987, 169, 73–74.
457. Singh, A. K., Kumar, D., and Rawlley, R. K., Bunseki Kagaku, 1984, 33, 499–502.
458. Wasey, A., Bansal, R. K., and Puri, B. K., Analyst, 1984, 108, 515–520.

459. Chen, X., Zhou, R., Wu, D., Dong, L., Beijing Shifam Daxue Xuebao Ziran Kexueban, 1982, 3, 94.
460. Bing, G., Jilin Daxue Ziran Kexue Xuebao, 1987, 3, 91–93.
461. Dhaneshwar, R. G., Palrecha, M. M., Zarapkar, L. R., Khasqiwale, K. A., and Radhakrishnan, T. P., in *First International Symposium on Trace Elements*, D. M. Sankar, ed., John Wiley and Sons, New York, 1983, pp. 93–101.
462. Feher, Z., Pungor, E., and Naray, M., Magyar Kem. Folyoirat, 1984, 90. 361–366.
463. Meng, F., and Zhao, Z., Fenix Hauxue, 1983, 11, 249–253.
464. Meng, F., and Zhao, Z., Wuhan Daxue Xuebao Ziran Kexueban, 1982, 4, 89–94.
465. Zang, S., Cathodic Stripping Voltammetry, Fenxi Ceshi Tongbao, 1987, 6, 26–29.
465a. Zlotkin, S., Can. Med. Assoc. J., 1985, 133, 1110.
466. Heinonen, J., *The Reliability of Radiochemical and Chemical Trace Analysis in Environmental Materials*, Technical Research Centre of Finland, Publication 22, Espoo, 1977.
467. anonymous, Quality Assurance in Biomedical Neutron Activation Analysis, IAEA-TECDOC-323, International Atomic Energy Agency, Vienna, 1984.
468. M'Baku, S. B., "Invitation to Participate in an IAEA Co-ordinated Research Programme," appendix 3, "Analytical Quality Assurance," International Atomic Energy Agency, June, 1983.
469. Muramatsu, Y., and Parr, R. E., *Survey of Currently Available Reference Materials for Use in Connection with the Determination of Trace Elements in Biological and Environmental Materials*, Report IAEA/RL/128, International Atomic Energy Agency, Vienna, 1985.
470. Okamoto, K., NIES, personal communication, November, 1985.
471. Suzuki, S., Okada, Y., Matumoto, K., and Hirai, S., Bull. Atomic Energy Res. Lab. Musashi Inst. Technol., June, 57–63, 1985.
472. M'Baku, S. B., and Parr, R. E., "Interlaboratory Study of Trace and Other Elements in the IAEA Powdered Human Hair Reference Material, HH-1," 6th International Conference on Modern Trends in Activation Analysis, Toronto, June, 1981.
473. M'Baku, S. B., and Parr, R. E., J. Radioanal. Chem., 1982, 69, 171–180.
474. Coetzee, P. P., and Pieterse, H., S. Afr. J. Chem., 1986, 39, 85–88.
475. Rains, T. C., NBS, personal communication, February, 1980.
476. anonymous, *Activation Analysis of Hair as an Indicator of Contamination of Man by Environmental Trace Element Pollutants*, Report IAEA/RL/50, International Atomic Energy Agency, Vienna, 1978.
477. Jenkins, D. W., *Toxic Trace Elements in Mammalian Hair and Nails*, EPA-600/4-79-049, U.S. Environmental Protection Agency, Las Vegas, 1979.
478. Iyengar, G. V., *Concentrations of 15 Trace Elements in Some Selected Adult Human Tissues and Body Fluids of Clinical Interest from Several Countries: Results from a Pilot Study for the Establishment of Reference Values*, Report No. 1874, Kernforschungsanlage Julich, Julich, 1985.
479. Matsubara, J., University of Tokyo, personal communication, 1984.
480. Luderitz, P., Marquardt, D., Leppin, S., Grosser, J., and Belakovsky, M. S., Z. Klin. Med., 1985, 20, 1515–1520.
481. Marlowe, M., Moon, C., Errera, J., and Stellern, J., Orthomolec. Psych., 1983, 12, 26–33.
482. Kamakura, M., Japan J. Hyg., 1983, 38, 823–838.
483. Ward, N. L., Spyrou, N. M., and Damyanova, A. A., J. Radioanal. Nucl. Chem., 1987, 114, 125–135.
484. Gibson, R. S., and Gibson, I. L., Sci. Total Environ., 1984, 39, 93–101.
485. Mederios, D. M., Mazhar, A., Burnett, E. W., Nutr. Res., 1987, 7, 1109–1115.
486. Houtman, J. P. W., Bos, A., Vis, R., Cookson, J. A., and Tjioe, P. S., J. Radioanal. Chem., 1982, 70, 191–208.
487. Vis, R. D., annex 10, IAEA Report for the 3rd RCM on the Significance of Hair Mineral Analysis as a Means for Assessing Body Burdens of Elemental Pollutants, Amsterdam, July, 1987.
488. Tykva, R., Vesely, J., Merta, A., and Votruba, I., annex 9, IAEA Report for the 3rd RCM on the Significance of Hair Mineral Analysis as a Means for Assessing Body Burdens of Elemental Pollutants, Amsterdam, July, 1987.

489. Matsubara, J., Ohomori, S., and Satoh, T., annex 8, IAEA Report for the 3rd RCM on the Significance of Hair Mineral Analysis as a Means for Assessing Body Burdens of Elemental Pollutants, Amsterdam, July, 1987.
490. Maugh, T. H., Science, 1978, 202, 1271–1273.
491. Stephens-Newsham, L. G., Duke, M. J. M., Overton, T. R., and Ng, D., J. Radioanal. Nucl. Chem., 1987, 113, 495–500.
492. Smith, B. L., Trace Element Med., 1987, 4, 131–133.
493. Muramatsu, Y., introduction, IAEA Report for the 1st RCM on the Significance of Hair Mineral Analysis as a Means for Assessing Body Burdens of Elemental Pollutants, Vienna, March, 1984.
494. Baumgartner, A. M., and Jones, P. F., "Radioimmunoassay of Hair for Determination of Drug Abuse Histories," 1979 Pacific Coast Conference on Chemistry and Spectroscopy, Pasadena, October, 1979.
495. Puschel, K., Thomasch, P., and Arnold, W., Forensic Sci. Internat., 1983, 21, 181–186.

Index

A

Acrodermatitis enteropathica, 50
Age
  trace elements and, 20–21
Age-dependent reference ranges, 108
Aluminum, 40
Amino acids, 7, 9
Ammonium pyrrolidine dithiocarbamate
    (APDC), 88–89
Anagen stage of hair growth, 9–10, 12
Anatomical location of hair, 19–20, 73–74
Anemia, 29
Animal experiments
  cadmium and, 42–43
  indications from, 43
  mercury and, 43
Anodic stripping voltammetry (ASV), 85, 94
Antimony, 26, 40
Arsenic, 12–13
  nonoccupational exposure to, 67–69
  occupational exposure to, 62–63, 65
  poisoning, 41, 44–45
  toxic effects of, 40
  washing procedures on sampling, 79
Atomic absorption spectrometry (AAS), 73, 87–90
  compared with other procedures, 93

B

Beryllium, 40
Blacks, trace elements in hair of, 21
Blood, trace elements in, 3

C

Cadmium, 20
  animal experiments with, 42–43
  nonoccupational exposure to, 66–68
  occupational exposure to, 63–64
  toxicity, 37–38, 40
Calcium
  and cystic fibrosis, 51
  and diet, 33
  and myocardial infarction, 56
  washing procedures on sampling, 79
Cancer, 53–54
Cardiovascular ailments, 57
Catagen stage of hair growth, 9, 10
Central nervous system (CNS)
  lead poisoning and, 40
  mercury poisoning and, 39–40
Certified reference material (CRM), 97, 101
Checklist, quality assurance, 98
Children
  chromium levels in, 2
  diabetics, 52
  environmental exposure to lead and mercury, 71
  iron-deficient, 29
  lead poisoning in, 12, 21, 39, 40, 45, 46
  zinc deficiency in, 29
Chlorine washing procedures, 79
Chromium, 2–3, 28
  and diabetes mellitus, 52–53
  occupational exposure to, 65
  toxic effects of, 40
Chrystotherapy, 26
Cleaning procedures for hair samples, 80–81, 83
"Club hairs," 9, 10
Cobalt, 29
  washing procedures on sampling, 79
Color of hair, trace elements and, 23–24
Commission of the European Communities
    (CEC), 89

Contraceptives, oral, and trace elements in hair, 25–26
Coordinated Research Programme (CRP), 80
Copper levels, 3, 13, 14, 17, 20, 22, 29, 50
  determining, 88, 90, 93
  effects of carcinoma on, 53–54
  hair color and, 23–24
  in identifying disease, 50–51, 52
  malnutrition and, 31–32
  normal ranges in, 107
  occupational exposure and, 62–63
  reactions to, 52
  toxicity and, 40
  washing procedures on sampling, 79
Cortex cells, 6, 7, 8
Cosmetic preparations, 14
Cuticle, 6–7, 8
Cystic fibrosis, 51

D

Dental health, fluoride and, 29
Dental profession, 2, 20, 61–62
Determining trace element levels, techniques for, 85–94
Diabetes mellitus, 52
Diabetics, chromium levels in, 2–3
Diagnostic aids, 60
Dietary supplements, 25, 113
Direct sample induction device (DSID), 93
Disease, role of trace elements in
  cancer, 53, 54
  cardiovascular, 57
  cystic fibrosis, 51
  diabetes mellitus, 52
  and diagnostic aids, 60
  hemodialysis, 57–58
  hypoglycemia, 52
  Kaschin-Beck disease, 55–56
  Keshan disease, 55
  mental, 60
  myocardial infarction, 56
  nonspecified, 54, 57
  reactions to copper and nickel, 52
  utilization of hair analysis data in, 113
Dissolving hair samples, 82, 83
Doctor's Data, Inc., 106
Drugs, hair analysis to detect use of, 113–114
Dye, hair, 14, 17

E

Electrothermal atomization techniques, 89
Endogenous trace elements, 12–13, 19

Environment, 19
  occupational, 44–46
  pollutants in, 2, 3, 11, 24, 65–71, 105
  rare minerals in, 13–14
  trace element pathways in, 15
Essential trace elements
  biochemical functions, 28
  classification, 27–28
  malnutrition and, 28
Exogenous trace elements, 13–14, 19

F

Facial hair, 19–20
Factors affecting trace elements
  age, race, and gender, 20–23
  anatomical location of hair, 19–20
  color of hair, 23–24
  diet and medicines, 25–26
  geographical location, 24–25
  length of hair, 17–19
Females, trace elements in hair of, 22
Fish, mercury-contaminated, 12, 24, 38–39, 46, 69–71
Fluorine deficiency, 29
Follicle, hair, 6–10

G

Gender, and trace elements in hair, 22
Geographical habitat, 24–25
Goiter, 29
Gold levels, 26
Growth, hair
  rates of, 10, 11, 74
  stages of, 9–10

H

Hair Analysis Standards Board, 15, 76, 81
Hair cycle, 8–10
  duration of stages in, 12
Hair shaft, 6, 8
Heavy metal concentrations (*see also individual elements*), 1–2, 13, 14, 41, 44
  exposure to, 62–63
  normal ranges, 106–109
  screening for, 112
Hematosiderosis, 49
Hemochromatosis, 49
Hodgkins disease, 57
Hypoglycemia, 52

I

Inductively coupled plasma atomic emission spectrometry (ICP/AES), 85, 92
　compared with flame AAS, 93
Industrialization, 24
Instrument calibration, 98–99
International Atomic Energy Agency (IAEA), 2, 75, 80, 92, 100, 107
Iodine
　deficiency, 29
　effect of cancer on levels of, 53–54
Iron levels, 22
　effect of cancer on, 53
　hair color and, 23
　toxic effects of, 40
Irradiation–decay–measurement cycles, 85–87
Itai itai byo, 37

K

Kaschin-Beck disease, 55–56
Keratinization process, 6, 10, 14
Keratoses, skin, 41
Keshan disease, 30, 33, 55

L

Lead
　levels, 2, 3, 12, 14, 20, 21, 22, 24
　nonoccupational exposure to, 66, 67, 68
　occupational exposure to, 64–65
　poisoning, 39, 40–41, 45–46
　toxic effects of, 40
　washing procedures on sampling, 79
Leaded gasoline, 39
Leishmaniasis patients, 26
Length of hair, 17–19
Lipid material in hair, 7
Livestock, nutritional status of, 33–35

M

Magnesium levels
　and cystic fibrosis, 51
　and hair color, 23
　and hypoglycemia, 52
Males, trace elements in hair of, 22
Malnutrition
　hair analysis to determine, 31–33, 36
　intrauterine, 31
　and manifestations of mineral deficiencies, 28–31
Manganese
　deprivation, 29–30
　determining levels of, 88, 90, 93
　nonoccupational exposure to, 67
　occupational exposure to, 67
　toxic effects of, 40
　washing procedures on sampling, 79
Measurement
　cycles, 85–87
　significance of, 4–6, 105–114
　techniques for, 85–94
Medicines, 25
Medulla cells, 6, 7, 8
Menkes syndrome, 26, 50
Mental disorders, 60
Mercury
　dentistry-related exposure to, 61–62
　levels, 1–2, 12, 14, 21, 24
　nondentistry-related exposure to, 64
　nonoccupational exposure to, 69–71
　poisoning, 38–40, 46
　toxic effects, 40
　washing procedures on sampling, 79
Mercury-contaminated fish, 12, 24, 38–39, 46, 69–71
Methyl isobutyl ketone (MIBK), 88–89
Minamata disease, 38–39
MineraLab Inc., 106–107
Mineral content, 7
Mining, exposure to heavy metals in, 62–63
Molybdenum deprivation, 30
Morphology, hair, 6–10
Murder of Napoleon, The, 37, 45
Myocardial infarction, 56
Myxedema, 29

N

National Institute for Environmental Studies (NIES), 100–102, 112
Neutron activation analysis (NAA), 1, 43, 73, 85–87, 90, 91
Nickel
　deficiency, 30
　levels, 3, 19
　reactions to, 52
Nutrition
　essential trace elements and, 27–28
　human and animal studies on, 31–36
　mineral deficiencies and, 28–31
　utilization of hair analysis data in, 113

O

Occupational environment, exposure to elements in
　arsenic, 44, 65

Occupational environment, exposure to elements in (*cont.*)
  cadmium, 37–38, 63–64
  chromium, 65
  dentistry-related, 2, 20, 61–62
  lead, 39, 41, 45, 46, 64
  mercury, 38–39, 61, 64
  mining-related, 62–63
  thallium, 65
  welding-related, 63

P

Parkinson's disease, 57
Pilocarpine iontophoresis sweat test, 51, 52
Pollutants, 2, 3, 11, 24, 65–71, 105
Pool model, 15
Pregnant women, zinc deficiency in, 31–32
Protocols, recommended sampling, 75–77
Proton-Induced X-Ray Emission (PIXE) spectrometry, 90–92, 107, 111
Psychemedics Corporation, 114
Public hair, 2, 20

Q

Quality assurance
  analyses, 96–98
  checklist, 98
  instrument calibration, 98–99
  and quality control, 99–100
  reference material, 100–103
  sampling, 96

R

Race, and trace elements in hair, 20–21
Ranges of trace element concentration, 105–109

S

Sampling
  anatomical location of hair, 73–75
  cleaning procedures, 80–81
  discoloring, 82
  quality assurance, 96
  recommended protocols, 75–77
  survey of procedures, 83–84
  washing procedures, 77–80
Scalp hair, 19, 21–23, 27
  age-dependent references ranges, 108
  copper and zinc concentrations in, 107
  sampling procedure, 74
Scalp medications, 13–14
Sebum, 8, 19, 20
Selenium levels
  effect of cancer on, 54

and Kaschin–Beck disease, 55
and Keshan disease, 33, 55
toxic effects of, 13, 40
washing procedures on sampling, 79
Silicon deficiency, 30
Skin bleach creams, 46
Spark source mass spectrometry (SSMS), 85, 92
  compared with AAS, 93
Standard reference material (SRM), 97, 101
Sweat, 8, 11, 15, 20
Systemic intoxication, 20
  clinical observations, 39–41
  consequences of elemental, 40
  toxic element in, 37–39

T

Techniques for determining trace elements, 85–94
Telogen stage of hair growth, 9, 10
Thallium
  occupational exposure to, 65
  poisoning, 47
  toxic effects, 40
Tin, 30
Tokyo Welfare Pension Hospital, 54

V

Vanadium levels, 30, 31
Vitamin B_{12}, 29

W

Washing procedures for hair samples, 77–80, 83
Water, 7, 9
  arsenic-contaminated, 12–13, 44, 69
Welding, exposure to heavy metals in, 63
Wilson's disease, 50

X

X-ray fluorescence (XRF) spectrometry, 82, 85, 90

Z

Zinc levels, 2, 13, 14, 19, 20, 21, 22, 24, 25, 27, 30, 51
  determining, 88, 90, 93
  effect of cancer on, 53–54
  hair color and, 23
  malnutrition and, 31–33, 36
  normal ranges in, 107
  nonoccupational exposure and, 66, 67, 68
  occupational exposure and, 62–63
  toxic effects on, 40
  washing procedures on sampling, 79